Urology

Editors

MARY ANNA LABATO
MARK J. ACIERNO

VETERINARY CLINICS OF NORTH AMERICA: SMALL ANIMAL PRACTICE

www.vetsmall.theclinics.com

March 2019 • Volume 49 • Number 2

ELSEVIER

1600 John F. Kennedy Boulevard ● Suite 1800 ● Philadelphia, Pennsylvania, 19103-2899

http://www.vetsmall.theclinics.com

VETERINARY CLINICS OF NORTH AMERICA: SMALL ANIMAL PRACTICE Volume 49, Number 2
March 2019 ISSN 0195-5616, ISBN-13: 978-0-323-67848-3

Editor: Colleen Dietzler

Developmental Editor: Meredith Madeira

Photocopying

Single photocopies of single articles may be made for personal use as allowed by national copyright laws. Permission of the Publisher and payment of a fee is required for all other photocopying, including multiple or systematic copying, copying for advertising or promotional purposes, resale, and all forms of document delivery. Special rates are available for educational institutions that wish to make photocopies for non-profit educational classroom use. For information on how to seek permission visit www.elsevier.com/permissions or call: (+44) 1865 843830 (UK)/(+1) 215 239 3804 (USA).

Derivative Works

Subscribers may reproduce tables of contents or prepare lists of articles including abstracts for internal circulation within their institutions. Permission of the Publisher is required for resale or distribution outside the institution. Permission of the Publisher is required for all other derivative works, including compilations and translations (please consult www.elsevier.com/permissions).

Electronic Storage or Usage

Permission of the Publisher is required to store or use electronically any material contained in this periodical, including any article or part of an article (please consult www.elsevier.com/permissions). Except as outlined above, no part of this publication may be reproduced, stored in a retrieval system or transmitted in any form or by any means, electronic, mechanical, photocopying, recording or otherwise, without prior written permission of the Publisher.

Notice

No responsibility is assumed by the Publisher for any injury and/or damage to persons or property as a matter of products liability, negligence or otherwise, or from any use or operation of any methods, products, instructions or ideas contained in the material herein. Because of rapid advances in the medical sciences, in particular, independent verification of diagnoses and drug dosages should be made.

Although all advertising material is expected to conform to ethical (medical) standards, inclusion in this publication does not constitute a guarantee or endorsement of the quality or value of such product or of the claims made of it by its manufacturer.

Veterinary Clinics of North America: Small Animal Practice (ISSN 0195-5616) is published bimonthly by Elsevier Inc., 360 Park Avenue South, New York, NY 10010-1710. Months of issue are January, March, May, July, September, and November. Business and Editorial Offices: 1600 John F. Kennedy Blvd., Ste. 1800, Philadelphia, PA 19103-2899. Customer Service Office: 3251 Riverport Lane, Maryland Heights, MO 63043. Periodicals postage paid at New York, NY and additional mailing offices. Subscription prices are $338.00 per year (domestic individuals), $662.00 per year (domestic institutions), $100.00 per year (domestic students/residents), $451.00 per year (Canadian individuals), $823.00 per year (Canadian institutions), $474.00 per year (international individuals), $823.00 per year (international institutions), and $220.00 per year (international and Canadian students/residents). To receive student/resident rate, orders must be accompanied by name of affiliated institution, date of term, and the *signature* of program/residency coordinator on institution letterhead. Orders will be billed at individual rate until proof of status is received. Foreign air speed delivery is included in all *Clinics* subscription prices. All prices are subject to change without notice. **POSTMASTER:** Send address changes to *Veterinary Clinics of North America: Small Animal Practice*, Elsevier Health Sciences Division, Subscription Customer Service, 3251 Riverport Lane, Maryland Heights, MO 63043. Customer Service (orders, claims, online, change of address): Elsevier Periodicals Customer Service, Elsevier Health Sciences Division Subscription **Customer Service 3251 Riverport Lane Maryland Heights, MO 63043. Tel: 1-800-654-2452 (U.S. and Canada); 314-447-8871 (outside U.S. and Canada). Fax: 314-447-8029. E-mail: journalscustomerservice-usa@elsevier.com (for print support); journalsonlinesupport-usa@elsevier.com (for online support).**

Reprints. For copies of 100 or more of articles in this publication, please contact the Commercial Reprints Department, Elsevier Inc., 360 Park Avenue South, New York, NY 10010-1710. Tel.: 212-633-3874; Fax: 212-633-3820; E-mail: reprints@elsevier.com.

Veterinary Clinics of North America: Small Animal Practice is also published in Japanese by Inter Zoo Publishing Co., Ltd., Aoyama Crystal-Bldg 5F, 3-5-12 Kitaaoyama, Minato-ku, Tokyo 107-0061, Japan.

Veterinary Clinics of North America: Small Animal Practice is covered in *Current Contents/Agriculture, Biology and Environmental Sciences, Science Citation Index, ASCA, MEDLINE/PubMed (Index Medicus), Excerpta Medica, and BIOSIS.*

Contributors

EDITORS

MARY ANNA LABATO, DVM
Diplomate, American College of Veterinary Internal Medicine (SAIM); Associate
Chair for Graduate Programs, Clinical Professor, Department of Clinical Sciences,
Cummings School of Veterinary Medicine, Tufts University, North Grafton,
Massachusetts, USA

MARK J. ACIERNO, MBA, DVM
Diplomate, American College of Veterinary Internal Medicine (SAIM); Professor,
Midwestern University, College of Veterinary Medicine, Glendale, Arizona,
USA

AUTHORS

MARK J. ACIERNO, MBA, DVM
Diplomate, American College of Veterinary Medicine (SAIM); Professor, Department of
Medicine, Midwestern University, Glendale, Arizona, USA

ALLYSON C. BERENT, DVM
Diplomate, American College of Veterinary Internal Medicine; The Animal Medical Center,
New York, New York, USA

STEPHANIE BORNS-WEIL, BA, DVM
Diplomate, American College of Veterinary Behaviorists; Assistant Professor, Department
of Clinical Sciences, Cummings School of Veterinary Medicine, Tufts University, North
Grafton, Massachusetts, USA

C. A. TONY BUFFINGTON, DVM, PhD
Diplomate, American College of Veterinary Nutrition; Veterinary Medicine and
Epidemiology, University of California, Davis, Davis, California, USA

KRISTINE ELAINE BURGESS, DVM
Diplomate, American College of Veterinary Medicine (Oncology); Associate
Professor, Department of Clinical Science, Cummings School of Veterinary Medicine,
Tufts University, North Grafton, Massachusetts, USA

EMMANUELLE BUTTY, DMV
Internal Medicine Resident, Cummings School of Veterinary Medicine, Tufts University,
North Grafton, Massachusetts, USA

JULIE K. BYRON, DVM, MS
Diplomate, American College of Veterinary Internal Medicine; Professor – Clinical,
Veterinary Clinical Sciences, The Ohio State University, Columbus, Ohio, USA

MIKEL DELGADO, PhD, CAAB
Veterinary Medicine and Epidemiology, University of California, Davis, Davis, California, USA

CAROL J. DeREGIS, DVM, PhD
Diplomate, American College of Veterinary Medicine (Oncology); Pieper Memorial Veterinary Center, Middletown, Connecticut, USA

MARILYN DUNN, DMV, MVSc
Diplomate, American College of Veterinary Internal Medicine; Fellow IR & IE, Professor, Centre Hospitalier Universitaire Vétérinaire, Faculty of Veterinary Medicine, University of Montreal, Saint-Hyacinthe, Quebec, Canada

MARY ANNA LABATO, DVM
Diplomate, American College of Veterinary Internal Medicine (SAIM); Associate Chair for Graduate Programs, Clinical Professor, Department of Clinical Sciences, Cummings School of Veterinary Medicine, Tufts University, North Grafton, Massachusetts, USA

MELISSA MILLIGAN, VMD
The Animal Medical Center, New York, New York, USA

TARA L. PIECH, DVM, MS
Diplomate, American College of Veterinary Pathologists; Clinical Assistant Professor of Clinical Pathology, Department of Pathology and Population Medicine, Midwestern University College of Veterinary Medicine, Glendale, Arizona, USA

YANN QUEAU, DVM
Diplomate, American College of Veterinary Nutrition; Research and Clinical Nutritionist, Research and Development Center, Royal Canin, Aimargues, France

JESSICA M. QUIMBY, DVM, PhD
Diplomate, American College of Veterinary Internal Medicine; Associate Professor, Department of Veterinary Clinical Sciences, The Ohio State University, Columbus, Ohio, USA

NATHALIE RADEMACHER, Dr Med Vet
Diplomate, American College of Veterinary Radiology; Diplomate of the European College of Veterinary Diagnostic Imaging; Associate Professor, Radiology, Veterinary Clinical Sciences, School of Veterinary Medicine, Louisiana State University, Baton Rouge, Louisiana, USA

CATHERINE VACHON, DMV, DVSc
Diplomate, American College of Veterinary Internal Medicine; Fellow IR & IE, Internal Medicine Clinician, Centre Hospitalier Universitaire Vétérinaire, Montreal University, Saint-Hyacinthe, Quebec, Canada

JODI L. WESTROPP, DVM, PhD
Diplomate, American College of Veterinary Internal Medicine; Professor, Department of Veterinary Medicine and Epidemiology, University of California, Davis, Davis, California, USA

KATHRYN L. WYCISLO, DVM, PhD
Diplomate, American College of Veterinary Pathologists; Clinical Assistant Professor of Clinical Pathology, Department of Pathology and Population Medicine, Midwestern University College of Veterinary Medicine, Glendale, Arizona, USA

Contents

 Video content accompanies this article at http://www.vetsmall. theclinics.com.

Incontinence is a frustrating condition for both pet owners and their veterinarians. Fortunately, most causes are easily diagnosed and most dogs respond to appropriate therapy. This article reviews normal urine storage and voiding, causes of incontinence, typical clinical presentation, diagnostics, and treatment.

Untreated house soiling presents a severe risk to the human–animal bond. Despite being one of the most common behavior problems reported to veterinarians, a majority of veterinarians surveyed reported a lack of confidence in their ability to diagnose nonmedical inappropriate elimination. Successful resolution depends on an appropriate diagnosis, which is arrived at by a thorough medical and behavioral history, once medical problems have been ruled out. A systematic approach to collecting history, noting clinical signs and ruling out differentials, is most likely to yield positive results in the shortest time.

Nephroliths are often clinically silent. When non-obstructive and of an amenable stone type, dissolution should be attempted. When problematic, nephrolithotomy can be considered. Depending on stone type, size, and species, extracorporeal shockwave lithotripsy or endoscopic nephrolithotomy are preferred techniques. Obstructive ureterolithiasis should be addressed immediately to preserve kidney function. Because of decreased morbidity and mortality and versatility for all causes, interventional techniques for kidney decompression are preferred by the authors. Proper training and expertise in these interventional techniques should be acquired before performing them on clinical patients for the best possible outcomes.

Dietary management of urolithiasis in dogs and cats is designed to dissolve calculi when possible and/or reduce the risk of recurrence. The diet must reduce urine relative supersaturation for the particular salt in order to prevent crystallization. To decrease urinary concentrations of crystal precursors, increasing water intake is essential regardless of the stone type. Altering the amounts of dietary precursors of the stone and controlling urine pH is mostly effective for struvite, urate, xanthine, and cystine, but still subject to controversy for calcium oxalate. The investigation of underlying metabolic disorders and close monitoring of animals at risk is recommended.

Cats that present with chronic lower urinary tract signs are often diagnosed with feline idiopathic/interstitial cystitis, a disease syndrome that is more than just a bladder disease and can be associated wtih a myriad of other co-morbidities. Further, gaining a better understanding of FIC (including the most accurate descriptive terminology) may help researchers, veterinarians, pet food companies, and clients develop and tailor the best possible approaches to management of these cat's unique health and welfare needs.

Urinary tract infection (UTI) is a common diagnosis in companion animal practice and is responsible for a significant proportion of antimicrobial use in veterinary medicine. The veterinary community has begun to follow the standards of care in human medicine and shift its definition of an UTI based on culture results and toward the presence of lower urinary tract symptoms. An improved understanding of the pathophysiology of UTI, risk factors for clinical disease, and the implementation of more reliable in-house diagnostic testing can lead to improved outcomes for patients and reduce inappropriate treatment. Investigation of antibiotic-sparing therapies holds some promise as well.

Stem cell therapy has tremendous potential for clinical application in the treatment of a variety of diseases in veterinary medicine. Based on the known desirable immunomodulatory properties of mesenchymal stem cells, this therapy has potential for treatment of a variety of renal diseases. This review details our current understanding of stem cell biology and proposed mechanism of action as applicable to renal disease. Studies performed in chronic kidney disease clinical trials and models of acute kidney injury are summarized with the goal of providing an overview of the current status of this treatment modality and its potential for the future.

A complete urinalysis is an essential diagnostic test to perform in veterinary patients. When interpreted in the context of a patient's clinical history, physical examination findings, and other diagnostic test results, a urine specific gravity, chemical analysis (often via semiquantitative dipstrip testing), and sediment examination are vital to detect both renal and nonrenal disorders. In this article, we describe the usefulness of each component of a urinalysis, the significance of and how to interpret results, and common causes of false-negative and false-positive results.

Cytologic evaluation of the urinary tract can be diagnostically rewarding in cases of renomegaly or when discrete kidney or bladder masses are identified. Cytology can often help to distinguish between cystic, inflammatory, and neoplastic disorders. Various types of cystic and benign urinary tract lesions, diseases associated with urinary tract inflammation, and the cytologic differences between primary and metastatic neoplasms of the kidney and bladder are described. Basic sampling techniques for urinary tract cytology are also discussed.

Urinary tract imaging is an important part of the diagnostic work-up in patients with urinary diseases. Multiple modalities are available, and this article provides an overview of the different modalities, techniques, and indications.

 Video content accompanies this article at http://www.vetsmall. theclinics.com.

Minimally invasive interventional therapies are the new standard of care in veterinary medicine. In comparison with standard surgical procedures, they are associated with minimal tissue injury, leading to shorter, smoother recovery and decreasing the perioperative morbidity and mortality. A thorough understanding of the therapeutic options available is essential to properly educate and inform clients. Proper equipment, technical expertise, and experience are essential prerequisites to many of these procedures.

Primary renal tumors are an uncommon diagnosis in small animals. Presentation, treatment, and prognosis depend on tumor type. Surgery with or without chemotherapy are the mainstays of treatment. Transitional cell carcinoma is the most common tumor of the urinary system. Clinical signs include hematuria, stranguria, and pollakiuria. Metastatic disease can develop over time within medial iliac lymph nodes, lungs, and vertebrae. Treatment of transitional cell carcinoma centers on chemo-therapy with mitoxantrone, vinblastine, or carboplatin. Other agents used with success, include toceranib phosphate and chlorambucil. Inter-ventional surgery, such as stenting and laser ablation, is used in a palliative setting addressing urinary obstruction.

VETERINARY CLINICS OF NORTH AMERICA: SMALL ANIMAL PRACTICE

SERIES OF RELATED INTEREST

Veterinary Clinics of North America: Exotic Animal Practice
https://www.vetexotic.theclinics.com/

THE CLINICS ARE NOW AVAILABLE ONLINE!
Access your subscription at:
www.theclinics.com

Preface

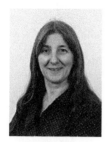 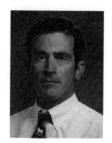

Mary Anna Labato, DVM, DACVIM (SAIM)   Mark J. Acierno, MBA, DVM, DACVIM (SAIM)
Editors

We are both very excited to have had the opportunity to edit this issue of *Veterinary Clinics of North America: Small Animal Practice*. There have been a number of publications over the years addressing concerns of the urinary tract, and our vision was to develop a concise and up-to-date reference that would be suitable for both the general practitioner and those working in more specialized areas of urology. This issue is the realization of that vision. We have tried to include practical information that can be implemented immediately as well as discussions of ongoing research in areas such as biofilm management and stem cell therapy. We have reached out to experts in the fields to present topics in urinary incontinence, inappropriate urinations, upper tract urolithiasis, nutritional management of urolithiasis, feline idiopathic cystitis, urinary tract infection, stem cell therapy, importance of urinalysis, urinary tract cytology, diagnostic imaging of the urinary tract, interventional therapies of the urinary tract, urologic oncology, and nutraceuticals for urinary tract use.

Perhaps the most humbling aspect of working on this issue was realizing how far we have come in the treatment of diseases of the urinary tract; however, at the same time, we understand that there is so much more to learn. Over the years, we have come to better understand the pathophysiology of urolith formation, yet we are still at the cusp of understanding how some stones are formed. We are starting to appreciate the genetics behind some urolith formation. We have developed ways to spare kidneys that would have been lost to ureteral obstructions. Relinquishment of dogs and cats for urinary incontinence and inappropriate urinations has decreased because there are now better management options. Diagnostic imaging of the urinary tract is multimodal, and the importance of urinalysis and cytologic examination has contributed to improvements in the management of developmental abnormalities, infection, and neoplasia. Owner recognition of the importance of diet and nutraceuticals in their own health has expanded into the veterinary profession so veterinarians must keep current on what is available for our companion animals.

We would like to thank those who have contributed to this issue, to whom we owe a debt of gratitude. They responded to a very short production deadline with good spirit and timeliness. It is an honor to have such colleagues. Their hard work has produced a

Vet Clin Small Anim 49 (2019) xi–xii
https://doi.org/10.1016/j.cvsm.2018.11.007
0195-5616/19/© 2019 Elsevier Inc. All rights reserved.

vetsmall.theclinics.com

reference that is suitable for readers interested in providing clinical cases the best possible care as well as those interested in the more advanced aspects of veterinary urology. We would also like to acknowledge the staff at Elsevier, especially Meredith Madeira, for all of their assistance and for keeping us on schedule.

Mary Anna Labato, DVM, DACVIM (SAIM)
Department of Clinic Sciences
Cummings School of Veterinary Medicine
Tufts University
200 Westboro Road
North Grafton, MA 01536, USA

Mark J. Acierno, MBA, DVM, DACVIM (SAIM)
Midwestern University
College of Veterinary Medicine
5715 West Utopia Road
Glendale, AZ 85308, USA

E-mail addresses:
mary.labato@tufts.edu (M.A. Labato)
macier@midwestern.edu (M.J. Acierno)

Canine Incontinence

Mark J. Acierno, MBA, DVM[a], Mary Anna Labato, DVM[b],*

KEYWORDS

- Incontinence • Urethral sphincter mechanism incompetence • Ectopic ureters
- Detrusor instability • Pelvic bladder

KEY POINTS

- Urinary incontinence is a frustrating condition to manage.
- Urinary incontinence may be from either a neurogenic or non-neurogenic cause.
- Medical management is often a viable option for non-neurogenic causes of urinary incontinence.
- Several interventional techniques have improved the treatment options for urinary incontinence.

 Video content accompanies this article at http://www.vetsmall.theclinics.com.

INTRODUCTION

At one time, dogs lived in the backyard and incontinence was not a serious issue; however, as dogs have moved into the home, the bedroom, and sometimes even owners' beds, the ability to control the timing of urination has become essential. As a result, incontinence has become a major source of frustration for affected dog owners and their veterinarians.

PHYSIOLOGY

The urinary cycle is divided into 2 distinct phases: the filling phase and the emptying phase.[1] The filling phase is dominated by the sympathetic nervous system. In this phase, the hypogastric nerve stimulates β-receptors in the body of the bladder and α-receptors in the trigone and proximal urethra, resulting in relaxation and stretching of the bladder and muscular constriction of the trigone and proximal urethra.[1,2] Thus, the body of the bladder acts as a relaxed reservoir, while the trigone region and the urethra act as a closed valve.

Disclosure Statement: The authors have nothing to disclose.
[a] Department of Medicine, Midwestern University, 5715 West Utopia Road, Glendale, AZ 85308, USA; [b] Cummings School of Veterinary Medicine, Tufts University, 200 Westboro Road, North Grafton, MA 01536, USA
* Corresponding author.
E-mail address: mary.labato@tufts.edu

Vet Clin Small Anim 49 (2019) 125–140
https://doi.org/10.1016/j.cvsm.2018.11.003
0195-5616/19/© 2018 Elsevier Inc. All rights reserved.

As the bladder becomes distended, stretch receptors in the wall of the bladder become stimulated and this information travels in the pelvic nerve to the spinal cord. Here it is relayed to the brainstem where the sensory information is integrated with conscious information from the forebrain.[1,2] When a decision to urinate occurs, an impulse to empty the bladder is carried down the spinal cord to the pelvic nerve that provides parasympathetic innervation to detrusor muscle fibers. This results in the simultaneous contraction of the bladder and relaxation of the trigone and urethra.[2] Areas of communication between adjacent muscle fiber membranes called tight junctions allow the contraction to spread quickly and evenly throughout the bladder.

Incontinence is the involuntary escape of urine during the storage phase of the urinary cycle. Clinically, this can present in different ways; however, the most common presentations are intermittent or continuous dribbling of urine combined with episodes of normal voiding. Causes of incontinence include urethral sphincter mechanism incompetence (USMI), ectopic ureters (EUs), pelvic bladder syndrome, detrusor instability, damage to the nerves controlling micturition, and primary neurogenic causes, such as a lower motor neuron bladder and overflow incontinence. In 1 older study of 563 dogs presenting with urinary incontinence, however, a vast majority were diagnosed with either USMI or EUs.[3]

HISTORY AND CASE WORK-UP

A detailed history is essential to differentiate incontinence from nocturia, pollakiuria, polyuria, and behavioral issues, all of which can be confused by owners for incontinence. Questions should focus on timing, volume, and events surrounding the leakage of urine. Helpful information includes whether the urination occurs when sleeping or if the dog dribbles continuously. Perhaps the "accidents" only occur at night and the owner has never actually witnessed them, suggesting possible nocturia or pollakiuria. In a case referred to one of the authors, the "incontinence" occurred when the dog met new people and was accompanied by rolling on her back, clearly indicating a behavioral issue.

A thorough physical, including a neurologic examination, should be performed. The genitals should be carefully examined for moisture, staining of the fur, and skin scalding, because an animal that is truly incontinent should have at least some of these signs. The genitals should be carefully examined to ensure they appear anatomically correct. It is important to ask owners to not allow their pet to void just prior to their appointment. Assessing the ability of the animal to normally urinate is important in ruling out retention micturition disorders, such as reflex dyssynergia, as well as bladder contractility disorders.

The importance of the neurologic examination cannot be overemphasized. Spinal cord conditions affecting L5 and above classically produce involuntary, erratic, reflexive emptying of the bladder with increased resistance of the external sphincter. Manual expression of the bladder is exceptionally difficult. In most cases, these dogs have significant neurologic deficits that make them easy to diagnose. Lesions of the sacral spinal cord can be subtle and require careful evaluation. These lesions can prevent bladder sensation from the pelvic nerve from traveling to the brainstem. As a result, the bladder can become overdistended while the patient makes no conscious attempts to urinate. These lesions also cause pudendal nerve dysfunction, resulting in decrease or loss of external sphincter resistance. An easily expressed bladder in a dog with no obvious neurologic deficits should raise the suspicion that a sacral lesion is involved.

Laboratory data should include a complete blood cell count, serum chemistry, and urine analysis with aerobic culture. The blood work helps rule out systemic diseases that can be confused with incontinence, such as chronic kidney disease or diabetes mellitus, resulting in polyuria. Urine samples should be taken via cystocentesis or collected by sterile catheterization, because free-catch urine does not yield reliable results. Urine analysis is important because it may implicate cystitis as a cause of the incontinence; however, the urine analysis should not be used to diagnose urinary tract infections (UTIs). The urine must be cultured and any antimicrobial therapy should be based on sensitivity results. Urine culture results can be difficult to interpret because UTIs can cause urge incontinence, but UTIs also are common with some anatomic abnormalities, such as EUs and urethrorectal fistulas. Further diagnostics are always indicated when incontinence does not resolve with appropriate antibiotic therapy.

URETHRAL SPHINCTER MECHANISM INCOMPETENCE

USMI is generally recognized as the most common cause of canine incontinence. Although infrequently described in neutered male dogs[4] or intact members of both genders, it has been reported to affect between 3.0% and 20.0% of all female spayed dogs.[5–9] Although incontinence can occur any time, clinical presentation typically is seen 3 years to 4 years after an uneventful ovariohysterectomy.[10] Classically, owners describe a dribbling of urine that is most noticeable when the animal is asleep.[11] Although commonly referred to as spay-related incontinence, the mechanism by which surgical ovariohysterectomy results in clinical incontinence is not clear. Historically it had been believed that because estrogen exerts a permissive effect on the α-receptors of the urethral sphincter, loss of estrogen decreased responsiveness to sympathetic stimulation resulting in diminished tone. More recently, elevations of gonadotropin-releasing hormone and luteinizing hormone resulting from loss of gonadal feedback[12–14] have been implicated in decreasing smooth muscle contractility in the lower urinary tract. In addition, it has been shown that spayed female dogs have an increased composition of collagen in their urinary tract and this may also contribute to incontinence.[15] Further complicating the issue, surgical manipulation of the urethra and bladder with suburethral slings has been shown to restore continence in some dogs,[16,17] suggesting that the actual cause of USMI is likely both complex and multifactorial.

There has been concern that spaying at an early age may be associated with the development of USMI, with various studies providing conflicting guidance.[6,18–21] Adding to the confusion, a systematic review suggests that some of these studies had issues in methodology, which could render their conclusions suspect.[22] Recently, a study has suggested that in dogs whose expected adult body weight is greater than 25 kg, there is an association with early neutering and USMI; therefore, spaying these dogs should be delayed until later in their first year.[10] No such association was found in smaller breed dogs. Additional research is needed in this area.

Although definitive diagnosis of USMI requires urodynamic testing, such equipment is only available at select referral institutions and, therefore, reserved for atypical or refractory cases. The urethra pressure profile can be helpful in diagnosing USMI in uncharacteristic patients. To perform this test, a specialized catheter that is capable of measuring pressure is inserted into the bladder of a sedated dog. Then, a computer-controlled motor slowly pulls the catheter out of the urethra while pressure is measured in the bladder, along the length of the bladder neck, and in the urethra. When finished, the computer generates pressure curves and determines both the urethral closure pressure and functional urethral length.[23] These pressure graphs allow the clinician to determine not only whether the pressure exerted by the urethral sphincter is adequate but whether the length of the functional urethra is normal (**Fig. 1**).

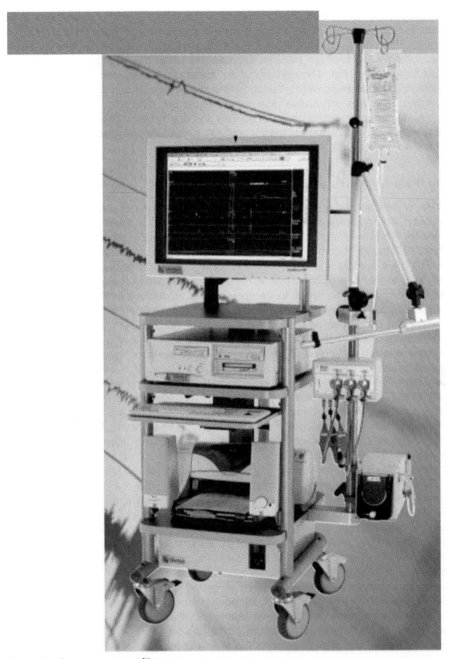

Fig. 1. Urethra pressure profile.

Given the prevalence, typical presentation, and the relative safety of the drugs used to treat USMI, diagnosis is often made empirically. In the Untied States, there are currently 2 commercially available Food and Drug Administration (FDA)–approved products: phenylpropanolamine (Proin, PRN Pharmacal, Pensacola, FL) and estriol

(Incurin, Allivet, St Hialeah, FL). Phenylpropanolamine is a nonselective adrenergic agonist that significantly increases urethral tone.[24,25] Potential side effects include hypertension, restlessness, irritability, tachycardia, increased intraocular pressure, and hepatic glycogenolysis.[26,27] Therefore, benefit of using this drug in patients with hypertension, diabetes mellitus, or glaucoma must be weighed against the potential risks. All patients should have their blood pressure checked before and then shortly after starting phenylpropanolamine.[27] Although rare, the authors have had clinical cases of normotensive animals becoming hypertensive after starting this medication. Treatment with phenylpropanolamine can be expected to result in resolution of clinical signs in 85% of USMI patients.[24,28] Due to its potential use in the manufacture of illicit substances, some states (eg, Arkansas, Iowa, Illinois, Louisiana, and Oregon) treat phenylpropanolamine as a controlled substance. Check local laws should be checked before dispensing.

In 2011, the FDA approved estriol (Incurin), a natural estrogen for the treatment of USMI in dogs. Estrogens work by exerting a permissive effect on the α-receptors of the urethral sphincter, thus increasing responsiveness to the sympathetic nervous system, resulting in increased urethral tone. Incidence of adverse effects seems low and mostly related to signs of estrus (swollen vulva and vulvovaginitis) and gastrointestinal upset (anorexia and vomiting). There is no evidence of bone marrow suppression even at high doses. Approximately 80% of dogs demonstrate improvement[29] with estriol treatment as a sole therapy ,and antidotal evidence suggests that it can be used with phenylpropanolamine for synergistic effects (**Table 1**).

In a small percentage of patients, medical management is unable to restore continence. Fortunately, several procedures exist. The least invasive involves endoscopic injection of a bulking agent into the urethral submucosa.[30–33] The effect is to stretch the urethral muscle fibers and narrow the urethral lumen, allowing for more effective urethral sphincter closure; 66% to 68% of dogs treated with this method attained full urinary continence after the procedure, whereas 46% to 60% of those that did not were able to achieve continence with addition of medical management.[30,33] The primary limitation of this procedure seems to be its temporary nature because dogs return to incontinence over time. In 1 study, dogs that achieved complete continence maintained that state for an average of 16.4 months whereas those that needed medical support after injection returned to incontinence in only 5.2 months.[33] Nevertheless, client satisfaction was universally high[33–35] (**Table 2**, Video 1).

Surgical placement of a hydraulic urethral occluder is another option for incontinent dogs that fail medical management. This is a newer procedure in which a silicone cuff is placed around the proximal urethra. The device is connected to an injection port, which is implanted in the subcutaneous tissue in either the medial aspect of the proximal thigh or along the ventral abdomen. The cuff provides increased urethral support while allowing the dog to urinate normally. Adding or removing saline from the injection port adjusts the amount of pressure the cuff exerts on the urethra, allowing for individual adjustments to be made for the specific patient (**Fig. 2**). A retrospective study of 27 dogs with urethral occluders showed excellent results, although 2 dogs did develop significant complications (seroma formation at surgical site, infection, worsening of incontinence, stranguria, partial to complete urethral obstruction secondary to adhesion or stricture formation).[36]

The hammock theory is commonly used to explain stress incontinence in women. This theory assumes that weakening of the anatomic structures responsible for maintaining correct anatomic orientation of the urethra and bladder allows for abdominal pressure to exert greater force on the bladder than the urethra allowing for urine to be expelled. Good success has been achieved in human medicine using a minimally

Table 1
Pharmacologic agents used in treatment of disorders urinary incontinence

Agent	Action	Dosages	Adverse Effects	Contraindications
Baclofen	Skeletal muscle relaxant	Dog: 1–2 mg/kg PO q8h	Weakness, pruritus, GI upset	
Bethanechol	Parasympathomimetic	Dog: 5–25 mg PO q8h	Vomiting, anorexia, cramping, ptyalism	Urethral obstruction, GI disease, hyperthyroidism
Dantrolene	Skeletal muscle relaxant	Dog: 1–5 mg/kg PO q8–12h	Weakness, GI upset, sedation, hepatotoxicity	Cardiopulmonary disease
Diazepam	Benzodiazepine, skeletal muscle relaxant	Dog: 2–10 mg/dog PO q8h	Sedation, polyphagia, paradoxic excitement, hepatotoxicity	Hepatic disease, pregnancy
Diethylstilbesterol	Reproductive hormone	Dog: 0.1–1.0 mg/dog q24h for 3–7 d then taper to once weekly	Estrus Behavioral change Myelosuppression Pyometra in intact females	Males Cats Pregnancy
Dicyclomine	Anticholinergic	Dogs: 5–10 mg/dog PO q8h	Sedation Dry mouth Urinary retention GI upset	Glaucoma GI obstruction Renal or hepatic disease Cardiac arrhythmias Hypertension
Ephedrine	α-Agonist	Dogs: 1–1.5 mg/kg PO q12–24h	Hypertension Inappetence	Hypertension Cardiac disease
Estriol	Reproductive hormone	Dogs: 2 mg PO q24h/14 d, then 1 mg q24h/14 d, then 0.5 mg q24h or to lowest effective dose	Less common than DES: Estrus Behavioral change Myelosuppression Pyometra in intact females	(Same as for DES) Males Cats Pregnancy
Flavoxate	Anticholinergic	Dogs: 100–200 mg/dog PO q12–24h	Sedation Dry mouth Urinary retention Gastrointestinal upset	Glaucoma Gastrointestinal obstruction Renal or hepatic disease Cardiac arrhythmias Hypertension

Drug	Mechanism	Dosage	Side Effects	Contraindications
Imipramine	Neuronal; uptake blocker Antimuscarinic	Dogs: 5–10 mg/dog orally q8h	Sedation Dry mouth GI retention GI upset Behavior changes	Seizure disorders, glaucoma Use of other anticholinergic or CNS depressants GI upset Cardiac arrhythmias Renal or hepatic disease
Phenylpropanolamine	α-Agonist	Dogs: 1–1.5 mg/kg PO q12–24h Cats: 1–1.5 mg/kg PO q12–24h	Hypertension Inappetance	Hypertension Cardiac disease
Phenoxybenzamine	α-Antagonist, urethral smooth muscle relaxant	Dog: 0.25 mg/kg PO q12–24h, or 2.5–20 mg/dog PO q12–24h	Hypotension, GI upset, tachycardia	Cardiac disease, glaucoma, diabetes mellitus, kidney failure
Prazosin	Same as phenoxybenzamine	Dog: 1 mg/15 kg PO q8h	As for phenoxybenzamine	As for phenoxybenzamine
terazosin	Same as phenoxybenzamine	Dog: 0.5–5 mg/dog PO q12–24h	As for phenoxybenzamine	As for phenoxybenzamine
Testosterone cypionate	Reproductive hormone	2.2 mg/kg IM q4–6wk	Behavioral change Perianal ademona Perineal hernias Prostatic disease aggression	Cardiac, renal, or hepatic disease

Abbreviations: CNS, Central Nervous System; DES, Diethylstilbesterol; GI, gastrointestinal; IM, intramuscular.

Table 2		
Sources of urethral bulking agents		
Macroplastique	Cogentix, Minnetonka, MN; Westborough, MA	www.cogentixmedical.com
Coaptite	Boston Scientific, Marlborough, MA	www.bostonscientific.com
Durasphere	Coloplast, Minneapolis, MN	www.coloplast.us
Collagen ReGain	Avalon Medical, Stillwater, MN	http://avalonmed.com

invasive procedure involving vaginal placement of a suburethral sling; however, complications are not uncommon.[37] Recently, studies have described techniques for using transobturator tape slings for the treatment of USMI in dogs.[16,17] Although good results have been reported, this procedure has yet to gain wide spread acceptance.

Medical treatment of USMI in male dogs is similar but less rewarding than treatment of their female counterparts. Only 44% of incontinent male dogs improve with administration of phenylpropanolamine.[4] Testosterone alone or in combination with α-agonists may improve continence; however, in 1 case series, only 38% of testosterone treated dogs became completely continent whereas 50% showed no response.[38] In addition, use of testosterone may be associated with serious side effects, including aggression and prostatomegaly.[4] For dogs that do not respond to medical management, endoscopic injection of a bulking agent and hydraulic urethral occluders are options.

ECTOPIC URETERS

EUs are an anatomic abnormality characterized by ureters that terminate and empty somewhere other than the trigone of the bladder. Embryologically, EUs are believed to develop as a result of abnormal growth and development of mesonephric and metanephric duct systems resulting in abnormal ureteral tube termination.[39]

Based on their point of attachment and behavior, EUs are divided into 2 categories: intramural and extramural. More than 95% of EUs are reported to be intramural in that the ureters attach to the bladder, tunnel below the submucosa, and open into the urethra or vagina.[40–42] Extramural EUs, which are rare, attach and empty directly into the

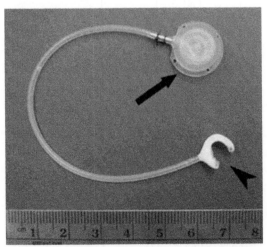

Fig. 2. Image of a urethral occluder. Arrow: subcutaneous access port; arrowhead: occluder.

urethra, vagina, or uterus. EUs occur bilaterally in 32% to 91% of cases and concurrent congenital abnormalities of the urogenital tract are common.[43-45] Studies have identified an increased incidence in certain breeds, including border terriers, briards, bulldogs, Entlebucher mountain dogs, fox terriers, golden retrievers, griffons, Labrador retrievers, miniature and toy poodles, Newfoundland dogs, Siberian huskies, Skye terriers, and West Highland white terriers[46-48]; however, EUs can occur in any breed. Classically described as a condition of young females with a history of dribbling urine since birth, dogs diagnosed later in life have been described in both genders.[43,49] Nevertheless, more than 90% percent of canine EUs are reported to occur in young female dogs.[43,48] A common scenario that the authors have encountered is that of a young female dog that has been surrendered to a shelter under false pretexts (ie, owner moving to new apartment and could not keep dog) that is noted to dribble urine when adopted.

Diagnosis of EUs has traditionally been performed using radiographic studies, including excretory urography and pneumocystography; however, these studies can correctly identify only approximately 78% of EUs .[45,50] Ultrasonography is another diagnostic imaging modality has been useful in the diagnosis of EU; however, its sensitivity and specificity has not been proved superior to traditional radiographic studies.[51] Recently, use of CT imaging for the diagnoses of EU has been described[50,52,53]; however, its application is likely to be limited. Rigid cystoscopy has been shown to correctly identify 100% of EUs[45,50] and allows visual inspection of the ureteral orifice, bladder wall, urethra, and vagina. Studies comparing CT to cystoscopy have found cystoscopy superior.[45,50] In addition, because a vast majority of EUs are intramural and, in more than 95% of cases, the ureter can be repaired using minimally invasive laser ablation techniques during the same anesthetic event as the diagnosis (**Fig. 3**). This allows for superior outcomes to traditional surgeries,[54] with shorter time under anesthesia and lower client costs. CT may play a role in planning corrective surgery in rare cases of extramural EUs where laser ablation is not an option.

Because as many as 94% of dogs with EUs have abnormalities of the upper urinary tract and/or lower urinary tract.[43,55] preprocedural diagnostic should include an abdominal ultrasound. Hydronephrosis, hydroureter, and pyelectasia are common[43,50,55] and other structural abnormalities of the kidney have been described. In cases of a kidney significantly damaged and likely nonfunctional, the patient may be better served by nephrectomy.

Reported continence rates for female dogs treated with laser ablation range from 77% to 85%, although only approximately 50% of the dogs for which there are data were fully continent immediately after the procedure.[54,56] The remainder required additional therapies, such as medical management (10%), urethral bulking injections (6%), or placement of an urethral occluder (12%). In a smaller study, success for return to continence in male dogs with EU was reported as high as 100%.[57]

DETRUSOR INSTABILITY

Detrusor instability (hyperspasticity and overactive bladder) is a sudden urgency to urinate combined with an involuntary bladder contraction. Typical presentation includes pollakiuria, urgency, and incontinence.[58] Depending on the underlying etiology, detrusor instability is divided into urge incontinence and idiopathic detrusor instability.[58] Urge incontinence occurs when there is an underlying condition, such as infection, neoplasia, or uroliths, the presence of which stimulates involuntary bladder contractions. If an underlying condition cannot be identified, the sudden urgency to urinate is referred to as idiopathic detrusor instability. Therefore, the first step in

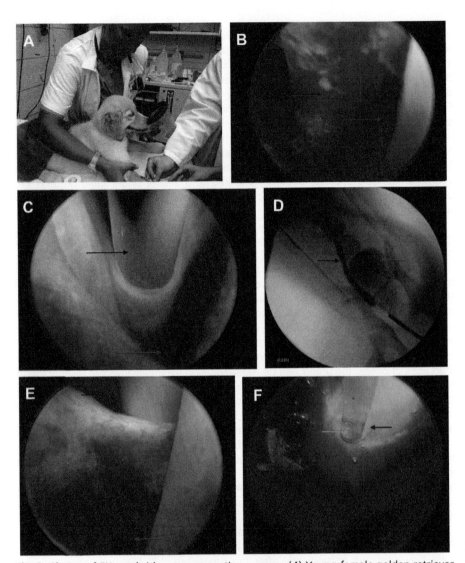

Fig. 3. Photos of EU urethrithoscopy correction surgery. (*A*) Young female golden retriever puppy whose foster family noticed near constant urine dribbling being prepared for cystoscopy (*B*) Where the opening to the urethra should be, there are 2 openings. Red arrow shows opening to urethra whereas black arrow points to opening of the EU. (*C*) Red arrow shows opening to urethra while black arrow points to guide wire, which is inserted in EU. (*D*) With a balloon catheter inserted in the EU, contrast is injected. Notice the EU highlighted (*black arrow*) against the bladder (*red arrow*). (*E*) EU with red rubber catheter inserted (*black arrow*); red arrow points to urethra. The red rubber catheter will be used for support when applying laser. (*F*) Tip of laser (*green arrow*) removing tissue separating EU (*black arrow*) from urethra. The red rubber catheter, which is difficult to see, is in the EU behind the black arrow.

working up a suspected case of detrusor instability should be to rule out any underlying conditions. Thorough physical and neurologic examination and history are essential. A cystocentesis should be performed and urine should be submitted for microscopic analysis and culture. An abdominal ultrasound should be performed with careful attention paid to the upper and lower urinary tracts. If an underlying condition is found, the first priority is to treat the condition.

Definitive diagnosis of idiopathic detrusor instability involves urodynamic testing.[58] Cystometrography involves inserting a catheter into the bladder and slowly inflating it with saline while monitoring intravesicular pressure. In dogs with idiopathic detrusor instability, the volume of fluid that can be infused before involuntary bladder contractions begin is dramatically reduced. Because this test requires specialized equipment that is only available at select referral institutions, cases are sometimes diagnosed based on clinical findings and response to treatment (**Fig. 4**).

Because bladder voiding is controlled by the parasympathetic nervous system, anticholinergic drugs can be effective in controlling the symptoms of detrusor instability.

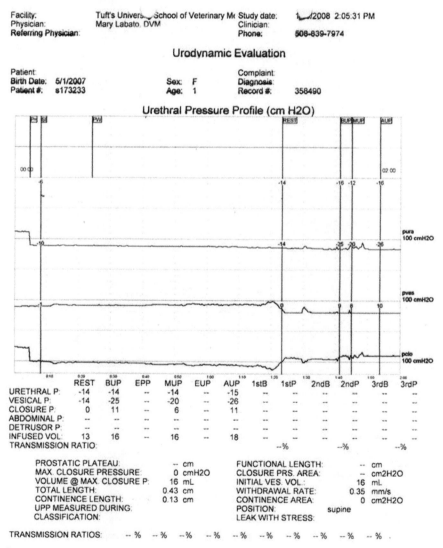

Facility:
Physician:
Referring Physician:
Tuft's University School of Veterinary Me
Mary Labato, DVM
Study date: 1/_/2008 2:05:31 PM
Clinician:
Phone: 508-839-7974

Urodynamic Evaluation

Patient:
Birth Date: 5/1/2007
Patient #: s173233
Sex: F
Age: 1
Complaint:
Diagnosis:
Record #: 358490

Urethral Pressure Profile (cm H2O)

	REST	BUP	EPP	MUP	EUP	AUP	1stB	1stP	2ndB	2ndP	3rdB	3rdP
URETHRAL P:	-14	-14	--	-14	--	-15	--	--	--	--	--	--
VESICAL P:	-14	-25	--	-20	--	-26	--	--	--	--	--	--
CLOSURE P:	0	11	--	6	--	11	--	--	--	--	--	--
ABDOMINAL P:	--	--	--	--	--	--	--	--	--	--	--	--
DETRUSOR P:	--	--	--	--	--	--	--	--	--	--	--	--
INFUSED VOL:	13	16	--	16	--	18	--	--	--	--	--	--
TRANSMISSION RATIO:							--%		--%		--%	

PROSTATIC PLATEAU:	-- cm	FUNCTIONAL LENGTH:	-- cm
MAX. CLOSURE PRESSURE:	0 cmH2O	CLOSURE PRS. AREA:	-- cm2H2O
VOLUME @ MAX. CLOSURE P:	16 mL	INITIAL VES. VOL.:	16 mL
TOTAL LENGTH:	0.43 cm	WITHDRAWAL RATE:	0.35 mm/s
CONTINENCE LENGTH:	0.13 cm	CONTINENCE AREA:	0 cm2H2O
UPP MEASURED DURING:		POSITION:	supine
CLASSIFICATION:		LEAK WITH STRESS:	

TRANSMISSION RATIOS: -- % -- % --% --% -- % -- % -- % -- % -- % .

Fig. 4. Cystometrography.

Oxybutynin (0.2 mg/kg orally very 8–12 h) or flavoxate hydrochloride (100–200 mg/dog orally every 6–8 h) is commonly recommended; however, dicyclomine (5–10 mg orally every 6–8 h) also may be efficacious.[59] There is some suggestion that the tricyclic antidepressant medication imipramine (5–15 mg orally every 12 h) may be helpful because it has anticholinergic effects and increases urethral closure pressure.

PELVIC BLADDER

Some dogs with significant urinary incontinence have a bladder that radiographically appears displaced caudally into the pelvic canal. Although usually associated with

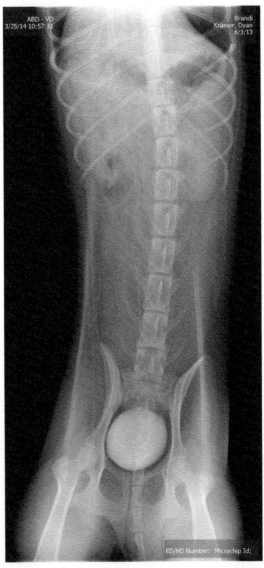

Fig. 5. Radiographic image of an overriding urethra and a pelvic bladder.

incontinence in large-breed female dogs, pelvic bladder incontinence has also been reported in male dogs.[60,61] The exact role that the position of the bladder plays is these dogs is not clear.[62] In people, the bladder neck and proximal urethra are normally within the abdomen so that increased abdominal pressure is applied equally to both the neck and body of the bladder maintaining continence. With a pelvic bladder, the neck and proximal urethra are outside the abdomen and these individuals experience only the increased pressure to the bladder. This can lead to leakage of urine. At least 50% of dogs whose bladder is located in the pelvis are completely continent.[60,62] In addition, there is little proof that in these dogs, the leakage of urine is associated with increased abdominal pressure. Lastly, dogs with pelvic bladder syndrome typically have a misshaped bladder that fails to taper at the junction with the urethra and have a shortened urethra with abnormal function and dysfunctional detrusor or a urethra that is over-riding the bladder (**Fig. 5**).[60,63] This suggests that pelvic bladder is actually part of a syndrome and is not solely dependent on the position of the bladder. Diagnosis is dependent on clinical signs and contrast radiography, which typically shows an abnormally shaped bladder that fails to taper at the junction with the urethra and is displaced caudally in the pelvic canal.[63] Treatment with phenylpropanolamine or estriol maybe helpful. In cases that are refractory to medical management, surgical implantation of a urethral occluder may be a helpful option.

Incontinent pets may be a continuous source of frustration to their owners as well as their veterinarians. For owners, stained carpets and bedding can quickly lead to aggravation with both pet and veterinarian. For veterinarians, the challenge is to find an optimum therapy that is medically and financially satisfying and maintainable. Fortunately, the most common causes of incontinence can be easily diagnosed and treated with a combination of medical management, minimally invasive procedures, and surgery.

SUPPLEMENTARY DATA

Supplementary data related to this article can be found online at https://doi.org/10.1016/j.cvsm.2018.11.003.

REFERENCES

1. Moreau PM. Neurogenic disorders of micturition in the dog and cat. Compend Contin Educ Pract Vet 1982;4:12–22.
2. Oliver JE, Lorenz MD, Kornegay JN. Disorders of micturition. In: Oliver JE, Lorenz MD, editors. Handbook of veterinary neurology. Philadelphia: WB Saunders; 1997. p. 73–88.
3. Holt PE. Urinary incontinence in dogs and cats. Vet Rec 1990;127:347–50.
4. Aaron A, Eggleton K, Power C, et al. Urethral sphincter mechanism incompetence in male dogs: a retrospective analysis of 54 cases. Vet Rec 1996;139:542–6.
5. Angioletti A, De Francesco I, Vergottini M, et al. Urinary incontinence after spaying in the bitch: incidence and oestrogen-therapy. Vet Res Commun 2004;28(Suppl 1):153–5.
6. Stocklin-Gautschi NM, Hassig M, Reichler IM, et al. The relationship of urinary incontinence to early spaying in bitches. J Reprod Fertil Suppl 2001;57:233–6.
7. Forsee KM, Davis GJ, Mouat EE, et al. Evaluation of the prevalence of urinary incontinence in spayed female dogs: 566 cases (2003-2008). J Am Vet Med Assoc 2013;242:959–62.

8. Thrusfeld MV, Holt PE, Muirhead RH. Acquired urinary incontinence in bitches: its incidence and relationship to neutering practices. J Small Anim Pract 1998;39: 559–66.

9. O'Neill DG, Riddell A, Church DB, et al. Urinary incontinence in bitches under primary veterinary care in England: prevalence and risk factors. J Small Anim Pract 2017;58:685–93.

10. Byron JK, Taylor KH, Phillips GS, et al. Urethral sphincter mechanism incompetence in 163 neutered female dogs: diagnosis, treatment, and relationship of weight and age at neuter to development of disease. J Vet Intern Med 2017; 31:442–8.

11. Krawiec D. Diagnosis and treatment of acquired canine urinary incontinence. Companion Anim Pract 1989;19:12–20.

12. Reichler IM, Hubler M, Jochle W, et al. The effect of GnRH analogs on urinary incontinence after ablation of the ovaries in dogs. Theriogenology 2003;60:1207–16.

13. Reichler IM, Jochle W, Piche CA, et al. Effect of a long acting GnRH analogue or placebo on plasma LH/FSH, urethral pressure profiles and clinical signs of urinary incontinence due to Sphincter mechanism incompetence in bitches. Theriogenology 2006;66:1227–36.

14. Donovan CE, Gordon JM, Kutzler MA. Gonadotropin-releasing hormone immunization for the treatment of urethral sphincter mechanism incompetence in ovariectomized bitches. Theriogenology 2014;81:196–202.

15. Coit VA, Gibson IF, Evans NP, et al. Neutering affects urinary bladder function by different mechanisms in male and female dogs. Eur J Pharmacol 2008;584: 153–8.

16. Claeys S, de Leval J, Hamaide A. Transobturator vaginal tape inside out for treatment of urethral sphincter mechanism incompetence: preliminary results in 7 female dogs. Vet Surg 2010;39:969–79.

17. Deschamps JY, Roux FA. Transobturator vaginal tape for treatment of urinary incontinence in spayed bitches. J Am Anim Hosp Assoc 2015;51:85–96.

18. de Bleser B, Brodbelt DC, Gregory NG, et al. The association between acquired urinary sphincter mechanism incompetence in bitches and early spaying: a case-control study. Vet J 2011;187:42–7.

19. Thrusfield MV. Association between urinary incontinence and spaying in bitches. Vet Rec 1985;116:695.

20. Spain CV, Scarlett JM, Houpt KA. Long-term risks and benefits of early-age gonadectomy in cats. J Am Vet Med Assoc 2004;224:372–9.

21. Howe LM, Slater MR, Boothe HW, et al. Long-term outcome of gonadectomy performed at an early age or traditional age in dogs. J Am Vet Med Assoc 2001;218: 217–21.

22. Beauvais W, Cardwell JM, Brodbelt DC. The effect of neutering on the risk of urinary incontinence in bitches - a systematic review. J Small Anim Pract 2012;53: 198–204.

23. Goldstein RE, Westropp JL. Urodynamic testing in the diagnosis of small animal micturition disorders. Clin Tech Small Anim Pract 2005;20:65–72.

24. Richter KP, Ling GV. Clinical response and urethral pressure profile changes after phenylpropanolamine in dogs with primary sphincter incompetence. J Am Vet Med Assoc 1985;187:605–11.

25. Byron JK, March PA, Chew DJ, et al. Effect of phenylpropanolamine and pseudoephedrine on the urethral pressure profile and continence scores of incontinent female dogs. J Vet Intern Med 2007;21:47–53.

26. Webster CR. Control of micturition: clinical pharmacology. Jackson Hole (WY): Teton NewMedia; 2001.

27. Carofiglio F, Hamaide AJ, Farnir F, et al. Evaluation of the urodynamic and hemodynamic effects of orally administered phenylpropanolamine and ephedrine in female dogs. Am J Vet Res 2006;67:723–30.

28. Scott L, Leddy M, Bernay F, et al. Evaluation of phenylpropanolamine in the treatment of urethral sphincter mechanism incompetence in the bitch. J Small Anim Pract 2002;43:493–6.

29. Mandigers RJ, Nell T. Treatment of bitches with acquired urinary incontinence with oestriol. Vet Rec 2001;149:764–7.

30. Barth A, Reichler IM, Hubler M, et al. Evaluation of long-term effects of endoscopic injection of collagen into the urethral submucosa for treatment of urethral sphincter incompetence in female dogs: 40 cases (1993-2000). J Am Vet Med Assoc 2005;226:73–6.

31. Wood JD, Simmons-Byrd A, Spievack AR, et al. Use of a particulate extracellular matrix bioscaffold for treatment of acquired urinary incontinence in dogs. J Am Vet Med Assoc 2005;226:1095–7.

32. Arnold S, Hubler M, Lott-Stolz G, et al. Treatment of urinary incontinence in bitches by endoscopic injection of glutaraldehyde cross-linked collagen. J Small Anim Pract 1996;37:163–8.

33. Byron JK, Chew DJ, McLoughlin ML. Retrospective evaluation of urethral bovine cross-linked collagen implantation for treatment of urinary incontinence in female dogs. J Vet Intern Med 2011;25:980–4.

34. Bartges JW, Callens A. Polydimethylsiloxane urethral bulking agent (PDMS UBA) injection for treatment of female canine urinary incontinence-preliminary results. Denver, CO: Proceedings of ACVIM Forum; 2011. p. 748–9.

35. Chew D. Diagnosis and managing urinary incontinence in dogs. Roanoke,VA: Proceedings of Virginia Veterinary Conference; 2015.

36. Reeves L, Adin C, McLoughlin M, et al. Outcome after placement of an artificial urethral sphincter in 27 dogs. Vet Surg 2013;42:12–8.

37. Nitti VW. Complications of midurethral slings and their management. Can Urol Assoc J 2012;6:S120–2.

38. Palerme JS, Mazepa A, Hutchins RG, et al. Clinical response and side effects associated with testosterone cypionate for urinary incontinence in male dogs. J Am Anim Hosp Assoc 2017;53:285–90.

39. Sutherland-Smith J, Jerram RM, Walker AM, et al. Ectopic ureters and ureteroceles in dogs: presentation, cause, and diagnosis. Compend Contin Educ Pract Vet 2004;26:303–10.

40. McLoughlin MA, Chew DJ. Diagnosis and surgical management of ectopic ureters. Clin Tech Small Anim Pract 2000;15:17–24.

41. Stone EA, Mason LK. Surgery of ectopic ureters: types method of correction, and postoperative results. J Am Anim Hosp Assoc 1990;26:81–8.

42. Dean PW, Bojarab MJ, Constantinescu GM. Canine ectopic ureter. Compend Contin Educ Pract Vet 1988;10:146–57.

43. Holt PE, Moore AH. Canine ureteral ectopia: an analysis of 175 cases and comparison of surgical treatments. Vet Rec 1995;136:345–9.

44. Reichler IM, Eckrich Specker C, Hubler M, et al. Ectopic ureters in dogs: clinical features, surgical techniques and outcome. Vet Surg 2012;41:515–22.

45. Cannizzo KL, McLoughlin MA, Mattoon JS, et al. Evaluation of transurethral cystoscopy and excretory urography for diagnosis of ectopic ureters in female dogs: 25 cases (1992-2000). J Am Vet Med Assoc 2003;223:475–81.

46. Holt PE, Thrusfield MV, Moore AH. Breed predisposition to ureteral ectopia in bitches in the UK. Vet Rec 2000;146:561.
47. North C, Kruger JM, Venta PJ, et al. Congenital ureteral ectopia in continent and incontinent-related Entlebucher mountain dogs: 13 cases (2006-2009). J Vet Intern Med 2010;24:1055–62.
48. Hayes HM. Breed associations of canine ectopic ureter: a study of 217 female cases. J Soc Adm Pharm 1984;28:501–4.
49. Thomas PC, Yool DA. Delayed-onset urinary incontinence in five female dogs with ectopic ureters. J Small Anim Pract 2010;51:224–6.
50. Samii VF, McLoughlin MA, Mattoon JS, et al. Digital fluoroscopic excretory urography, digital fluoroscopic urethrography, helical computed tomography, and cystoscopy in 24 dogs with suspected ureteral ectopia. J Vet Intern Med 2004; 18:271–81.
51. Lamb CL, Gregory SP. Ultrasonographic findings in 14 dogs with ectopic ureter. Vet Radiol Ultrasound 1998;39:218–23.
52. Anson A, Strohmayer C, Larringaga JM, et al. Computed tomographic retrograde positive contrast cystography and computed tomographic excretory urography characterization of a urinary bladder diverticulum in a dog. Vet Radiol Ultrasound 2018. [Epub ahead of print].
53. Fox AJ, Sharma A, Secrest SA. Computed tomographic excretory urography features of intramural ectopic ureters in 10 dogs. J Small Anim Pract 2016;57:210–3.
54. Berent AC, Weisse C, Mayhew PD, et al. Evaluation of cystoscopic-guided laser ablation of intramural ectopic ureters in female dogs. J Am Vet Med Assoc 2012; 240:716–25.
55. Mason LK, Stone EA, Biery DN. Surgery of ectopic ureters: pre- and postoperative radiographic morphology. J Am Anim Hosp Assoc 1990;26:73–9.
56. Berent AC. Advances in urinary tract endoscopy. Vet Clin North Am Small Anim Pract 2016;46:113–35.
57. Berent AC, Mayhew PD, Porat-Mosenco Y. Use of cystoscopic-guided laser ablation for treatment of intramural ureteral ectopia in male dogs: four cases (2006-2007). J Am Vet Med Assoc 2008;232:1026–34.
58. Lappin MR, Barsanti JA. Urinary incontinence secondary to idiopathic detrusor instability: cystometrographic diagnosis and pharmacologic management in two dogs and a cat. J Am Vet Med Assoc 1987;191:1439–42.
59. Lane IF. Use of anticholinergic agents in lower urinary tract disease. In: Bonagura JD, editor. Kirk's current veterinary therapy XIII: small animal practice. Philadelphia: WB Saunders; 2000. p. 899–902.
60. DiBartola SP, Adams WM. Urinary incontinence associated with malposition of the urinary bladder. Kirk's current veterinary therapy XIII: small animal practice. Philadelphia: WB Saunders; 1983. p. 1089–92.
61. Acierno MJ, Labato MA. Canine Incontinence. Compend Contin Educ Pract Vet 2006;28:591–600.
62. Mahaffey MB, Barsanti JA, Barber DL, et al. Pelvic bladder in dogs without urinary incontinence. J Am Vet Med Assoc 1984;184:1477–9.
63. Silverman S, Long CD. The diagnosis of urinary incontinence and abnormal urination in dogs and cats. Vet Clin North Am Small Anim Pract 2000;30:427–48.

Inappropriate Urination

Stephanie Borns-Weil, BA, DVM

KEYWORDS

- Inappropriate urination • Diagnosis • Dogs • Cats • Human–animal bond • Periuria

KEY POINTS

- Untreated house soiling presents a severe risk to the human–animal bond.
- Despite being one of the most common behavior problems reported to veterinarians, a majority of veterinarians surveyed reported a lack of confidence in their ability to diagnose nonmedical inappropriate elimination.
- Successful resolution depends on an appropriate diagnosis, which is arrived at by a thorough medical and behavioral history once medical problems have been ruled out.
- A systematic approach to collecting history, noting clinical signs and ruling out differentials is most likely to yield positive results in the shortest time.

Untreated house soiling presents a severe risk to the human–animal bond. Dog and cats that soiled the home were 2 to 4 times and 2 to 6 times, respectively, more likely to be relinquished to a shelter.[1–3] Those remaining in the home are at greater risk of death and poor welfare. Cats or dogs may be confined to the outside, where they face social isolation, predation, and automobile-related trauma. A weak human–animal bond is associated with less veterinary care, which impacts health and well-being.[4,5]

Despite being one of the most common behavior problems reported to veterinarians, a majority of veterinarians surveyed reported a lack of confidence in their ability to diagnose nonmedical inappropriate elimination. According to a survey, one-third of veterinarians were unable to correctly distinguish between urine marking and inappropriate toileting behavior in cats.[6] Whereas 73% of veterinary schools in the United States have instruction in animal behavior, it was a core requirement in less than one-half.[5] In the absence of formal training, most graduates rely on lay sources such as the Internet and television, rather than science-based publications.[7]

Inappropriate urination can be frustrating for veterinarians as well as clients. Successful resolution depends on an appropriate diagnosis, which is arrived at by a thorough medical and behavioral history once medical problems have been ruled out. A systematic approach to collecting history, noting clinical signs and ruling out

The author has nothing to disclose.
Department of Clinical Sciences, Cummings School of Veterinary Medicine at Tufts University, 200 Westboro Road, North Grafton, MA 01536 USA
E-mail address: stephanie.borns-weil@tufts.edu

Vet Clin Small Anim 49 (2019) 141–155
https://doi.org/10.1016/j.cvsm.2018.10.003
0195-5616/19/© 2018 Elsevier Inc. All rights reserved.

differentials, is most likely to yield positive results in the shortest time. The goal of this article is to provide up-to-date information that will facilitate the diagnosis and treatment of feline and canine periuria in the context of general practice.

A WORD ABOUT TERMINOLOGY

The challenge of diagnosing and treating inappropriate urination in dogs and cats is further compounded by an inconsistent and sometimes contradictory use of terminology in the veterinary literature. The terms inappropriate elimination and house soiling are used to describe all urination, including marking, that occurs outside of desirable locations by some authors. Other authors use the terms to refer only to nonmarking urination. For still others, the terms inappropriate toileting and latrine behavior are used to describe micturition rather than marking.[8,9] I use the following definitions for this article.

Inappropriate Urination, House Soiling, and Periuria

Inappropriate elimination, house soiling, and periuria are the general terms used describe all urine that is produced for any reason by cats and dogs in areas that are undesirable for their owners.

Marking

Urine marking in cats and dogs refers to the deposition of urine for the purpose of communication.

Spraying

Spraying describes a form of feline urine marking that involves a fixed action pattern. A spraying cat stands with an erect and twitching tail and releases a jet of urine against a vertical surface. It is often accompanied by treading of the hind feet.

Toileting

Inappropriate toileting refers to nonmarking micturition by cats and dogs outside of areas designated by the owners.

FELINE INAPPROPRIATE URINATION

For kittens, the purpose of urination is entirely physiologic, to eliminate metabolic waste. In the first weeks of life, urination and defecation are stimulated when the queen licks the kitten's perineum to stimulate elimination. At 5 to 6 weeks of age, kittens begin to urinate on their own and to move away from the nest area to eliminate.[10] They gravitate toward loose, litter-like substrates if they are made available.[11] When presented with the substrate, they also begin displaying species typical behavior sequence associated with urination typified by digging, sniffing, circling, squatting, and covering.[8,9] Although cats are drawn naturally to litter-like substrates, learning is also an important part of appropriate toileting. When kittens use the litter box to relieve themselves, they associate the relief of emptying a full bladder with the litter box, which reinforces its use.[8,12]

Once a cat reaches sexual maturity, urine has a behavioral as well as a physiologic function. Urine marking serves as an important means of communication between conspecifics along with bunting to deposit facial pheromones and scratching to create visual marks.

Inappropriate elimination is more common in multicat homes.[8,9,13] Cats are twice as likely to toilet inappropriately and 6 times more likely to mark if they live with 1 or more other cats.[9] Owners are often unaware which cat is responsible for the problem. There are many recommendations for identifying the culprit, all of which have limitations. One option is to separate the cats. However, if the cause of periuria is social stress between the cats, the problem may resolve without revealing the cat that was responsible. Fluorescein, which causes urine to fluoresce under black light, may be administered by mouth to the presumptive culprit. Urine stains are examined 24 hours later with a black light to reveal the presence of fluorescein. False positives are common because all urine fluoresces under black light, although the stains with fluorescein are brighter. Also, fluorescein may stain carpets and furniture.[10,14] The safest and most effective way of finding the culprit is to set up video cameras in areas of the house where urine is frequently found. If there are many soiled areas, the cats' access to the whole house can be restricted during video monitoring.

Is It Medical or Behavioral?

The first step is in the diagnostic process is to determine whether the problem is medical or behavioral. Even when the problem seems to be behavioral, this step should not be skipped. Because cats tend to hide illness, inappropriate elimination may be the only hint of a medical problem. Any disease process that causes pollakuria, stranguria, polyuria, or dysuria may trigger urination outside the litter box, including upper and lower urinary tract disease and metabolic conditions such as hyperthyroidism and diabetes mellitus. Medical conditions should be systematically ruled out with a full physical examination, urinalysis, urine culture by cystocentesis, complete blood count, serum chemistry panel, and thyroid testing in older cats. Uroliths and other abnormalities such as a space-occupying mass in the abdomen that may impair normal micturition should be ruled out with diagnostic imaging.[8,10,11,15–18] Feline idiopathic cystitis may be difficult to differentiate from behavioral periuria on the basis of laboratory results and history because both conditions may be precipitated by stress.[19] However, it is beyond the scope of this article to discuss feline idiopathic cystitis, about which there is a plethora of excellent scholarship.

Other medical issues that cause pain or reduced mobility may directly affect litter box use. For example, a cat with osteoarthritis may be unable or unwilling to use a box with high sides or at the top of a flight of stairs. House soiling is a common clinical sign associated with cognitive dysfunction syndrome. Gunn-Moore and colleagues[20] found that 35% of cats over the age of 11 years suffer from cognitive dysfunction syndrome.[15] Even when medical issues are found, the presence of a medical problem does not exclude the possibility of a comorbid behavioral etiology.[8,16]

Behavioral Periuria

Once a medical problem is ruled out, the next step is to use the behavioral history to characterize the behavioral problem. Multiple factors distinguish marking from inappropriate toileting. However, no single factor is sufficiently sensitive or specific to diagnosis an individual cat with either marking or toileting problems.[9]

The Behavioral History

Very specific information about the location (target objects or substrates, area of the house, vertical or horizontal surface) volume, and timing of inappropriate elimination should be collected. A thorough litter box history is also needed, including information about litter box husbandry, the number and location of boxes, the box style (covered vs open, high vs low sided, self-cleaning), litter type (clumping vs clay vs pearls; scented vs unscented). Cats may consider contiguous litter boxes as a single box, so the number of litter box locations may be more pertinent.[14] There is evidence that the social environment may be at least as important a contributor to both litter box problems and marking as the physical environment.[9,16] The number of adults and children in the home, the quality and quantity of interactions between the patient and family members, the daily schedule and amount of time the cat spends at home alone, the relationship between the patient and other animals in the home, and the presence of outdoor cats near the home are all important pieces of the puzzle. Changes in the environment such as a move, recent travel, schedule change, new baby, new roommate, and new appliances should be noted. Other behavioral problems such as aggression or fear are also relevant. A well-crafted questionnaire can be an invaluable tool for gathering lengthy histories. A customizable downloadable Cat Owner Questionnaire can be found in the American Association of Feline Practitioners/International Society of Feline Medicine Guidelines for Diagnosing and Solving House-Soiling and Behavior in Cats.[16]

Marking

The function of urine marking is to communicate information about a cat's sexual status and presence to conspecifics. Although undesirable when performed in the context of a house, urine marking is a normal feline behavior that occurs most frequently in males and in intact cats. However, if a female in estrus is nearby, male cats are more likely to spray regardless of neuter status.[21]

Marking also serves a territorial function, although it does not serve to deter intruders. Urine is deposited in core areas of a cat's territory, not at the boundaries. Chemosignals in urine allow cats move through a common space without encountering one another, thus avoiding potential conflict.[17,21]

Anxiety and environmental stressors also trigger urine marking, although the reason for stress marking is not well-understood. Marking may serve to build a cat's confidence by making the environment seem more familiar. Alternatively, marking may represent a displacement behavior. Intercat aggression is a common cause of stress marking that owners may not be aware of. Owners may not notice subtle agonistic interactions such as staring at or blocking the movement of a feline housemate. Other common stressors for indoor cats are insufficient mental stimulation and social isolation. Separation anxiety is commonly expressed as urine marking. Schwartz[22] noted that 75% of cats with separation anxiety urinate on their owner's bed.

Cats are more likely to deposit urine on vertical than horizontal surfaces when marking. Marked areas tend to be prominent places in the cat's core area and places with social significance. Windows and doors, corners and furniture legs, items associated with people or other animals in the home, and new items are common targets. There is no substrate preference associated with marking. Some authors propose that electrical objects such as toasters are marked because they generate heat, which presumably aids in spreading the scent.[8] Marking is not accompanied by premicturition and postmicturition behaviors such as digging and burying. Most cats stand rather than squat to mark. Unless there are comorbid toileting issues, marking cats continue to use a litter box to urinate and defecate.

Neutering is a very effective treatment for intact cats of both sexes. Gonadectomy was found to decrease spraying by 90% in males and 5% in females.[23] Territorial marking at doors and windows can be managed by blocking access to those areas and/or preventing outdoor cats from approaching the house. In warm seasons, motion-activated water sprayers may keep outdoor cats away. Bird feeders that also attract predatory outdoor cats should be removed. Feral cats should not be fed near the house. All urine marks should be cleaned and treated with an odor-mitigating product to prevent the patient from refreshing the marks as they fade.

In multicat homes, owners should be instructed about how to recognize signs of trouble between the cats. Advice about treatment for intercat aggression should be given if needed. In homes where cats are not socially bonded, an "environment of plenty" in which resources such as food, water bowls, and window seats are duplicated and spread throughout the home can defuse stress that is caused by forcing cats to congregate to meet their needs.[14] The Five Pillars of a Healthy Feline Environment offer valuable environmental guidelines for owners designed to decrease environmental stress and improve feline welfare by ensuring that a cat's home environment is safe from conflict with other cats and rich with social interaction and predatory play opportunities.[16,24]

Although marking is not associated with litter box problems, optimizing the litter box environment may contribute to a reduction in marking. Cleaning soiled areas with an enzyme solution, scooping daily and cleaning the box weekly resulted in a significant decrease in marking.[25]

Many studies support the use of Feliway synthetic feline facial pheromones to treat spraying and nonspraying marking. Pageat and Gaultier[26] reported a 96.7% decrease in recent onset marking with Feliway. A metaanalysis by Mills and colleagues[27] 2011 found treatment of urine marking with the synthetic analogue of F3 facial fraction pheromone therapy reduced spraying by more than 90%. Hunthausen[28] reported a decrease in the number of urine marks with Feliway but noted that two-thirds of the cats in the study continued to mark regularly after treatment.

Pharmacotherapy may be a very helpful component of treatment for urine marking. In a randomized, double-masked, placebo-controlled study, fluoxetine decrease the mean number of weekly urine marks from 8.6 to 0.4 in 8 weeks. A decrease in food intake was reported in 44% of the cats in the treatment group.[29] Clomipramine was also found to decrease urine spraying by 75% in 80% of cats.[30] Reported adverse effects include anticholinergic effects, gastrointestinal disturbance, and sedation, with sedation being the most common.[31] In a study by Hart and colleagues,[32] buspirone resulted in a 75% reduction of spraying and nonspraying urine marking in 55% of the cats treated. Better results were seen in homes with more than 1 cat. Diazepam decreased spraying in 55% of cats.[33] However, treatment with oral diazepam is no longer recommended because it has been associated with fatal acute hepatic necrosis.[34] A complete blood count and chemistry panel is advisable before initiating treatment. Because the medications are not labeled by the US Food and Drug Administration for use in cats, informed consent should be obtained from owners.

Inappropriate Toileting

Abnormal toileting is characterized by normal eliminatory behaviors performed in undesirable places. Cats that toilet inappropriately may or may not also use the litter box for defecation and/or urination. Those that urinate and defecate outside the box are more likely to be diagnosed with a toileting rather than marking problem.[21] Cats usually deposit urine on horizontal surfaces when voiding. Inappropriate toileting is generally accompanied by normal preeliminary and posteliminary behaviors, unlike marking. However, the behaviors are sometimes truncated. One study found that inappropriate toileting cats are less likely to cover their urine.[9] Another study found that they are less likely to dig in the litter before urinating.[35] Unlike marking, soiled areas have no social significance. Urine may be found in hidden areas such as under beds or next to the litter box.[8,10,14,16,18]

Motivations for inappropriate toileting can be divided into 2 main categories, namely, aversions and preferences. Any aspect of the toileting experience may be objectionable to cats with litter box aversion. Poor litter box hygiene is the leading cause of toileting problems.[14] The visual presence of waste in the box may be more averse than odor.[36] A cat may also object to the location, the type of box, and/or the type of litter. Aversion to the box can also be learned. A cat that was attacked by a feline housemate in the litter box or a cat with a history of stranguria or dysuria may be classically conditioned to fear and avoid the litter box.

Preferences also guide a cat's decision to eliminate inappropriately. A cat may prefer a location that is protected from other animals or young children. Alternatively, she may prefer a substrate that is more absorbent and less coarse than litter, such as clothing or bedding. Some cats are attracted to sinks and bathtubs to urinate because the waste disappears down the drain and leaves no visual trace.

The factors that maintain the behavior may be different from those that triggered it initially. A cat may object to a litter box that is not scooped for a weekend and begin urinating on the living room rug. She may then find that she prefers the new texture to that of the box. Even when the box is cleaned regularly again, she continues to choose the preferred substrate. Reasons for inappropriate elimination are frequently multifactorial, which further complicates the diagnostic process. A cat that lives with an aggressive feline housemate may be diagnosed with urine marking and feline idiopathic cystitis secondary to anxiety. She may also have developed an aversion to the litter box because she fears that she may be attacked while she eliminates.

Litter box hygiene should be optimized. Boxes should be scooped 1 to 2 times daily. Litter should be replaced and the boxes should be thoroughly cleaned with mild soap and water weekly. Old boxes should be replaced annually. The formula n + 1 boxes (1 box per cat + 1 box) is often cited as a guide for the number of litter boxes. In my experience, the number of boxes depends on many factors. For cats that are socially bonded, n + 1 may not be necessary. Owners who scoop and clean boxes more frequently may also be able to get away with fewer litter boxes. In contrast, more than n + 1 boxes may be required if owners scoop and clean infrequently. All soiled places must be cleaned thoroughly to remove every trace of odor. One study found that enzymatic cleaners were most effective at removing urine odor.[37] Zero Odor, a new nonenzymatic product has proven effective.[38]

Whether the cats prefer a covered or uncovered litter box may depend on the individual. Two studies demonstrated that most cats prefer uncovered boxes, although other studies have found that there is no general preference.[39,40] Uncovered boxes have the advantage of promoting better hygiene by making owners aware when a box needs scooping or cleaning.[8,16] Cats prefer large litter boxes.[39,40] Litter boxes should be 1.5 times a cat's length from nose to tail if a cat is to have adequate space to perform the preeliminatory and posteliminatory behaviors comfortably.[8] In a study of box preferences, cats were found to prefer boxes that are 86 × 29 × 14 cm, which is larger than a standard litter box.[40] For very large cats, owners may need to improvise by using a large plastic storage bin with an opening cut into the side. Tall-sided boxes and automatic self-cleaning boxes may not be acceptable to some cats.

Cats that eliminate near the box, attenuate preelimination and postelimination behaviors, or complete the eliminatory sequence outside of the box most likely have an aversion to the box or the litter.[35,41] Cats that balance on the sides of the litter box to eliminate usually object to the litter.[16] Litter is marketed to people, not cats. Because people object to the odor of feces and urine, many of the litters on the market are designed to mitigate the smell with baking soda or perfumes. Whereas some cats tolerate scented litter, most prefer varieties free of additives and scents.[41] They also prefer fine-grained, clumping, sandlike litter rather than course or pearl-like textures.[11,42]

Boxes should be placed in a quiet, private location where the cats will not be disturbed by other animals or young children.[8] Elderly or infirm cats may need a litter box that does not require the use of stairs to reach. Dogs can be kept away from litter boxes with a gate or by placing a hook and eye on the door to keep an opening large enough for a cat but not for a large dog. Social conflict may be a central reason why cats in multicat homes are more prone to inappropriate toileting as well as marking. Locations should be chosen that enable all cats to use the box without encountering other cats and to avoid other cats on the way to the litter box.[16] Care should be taken to avoid putting litter boxes near noisy appliances such as washers and dryers. One of my patients refused to use a litter box that we placed too close to a radiator that became uncomfortably hot in the winter months.

The optimal box and litter for an individual cat can best be determined by offering a variety of options. A buffet of litter boxes can be placed in each litter box station so that the cat can choose which is preferable.[14,18]

Although environmental and social stressors are usually associated with marking, they have also been shown to increase the risk of inappropriate toileting. A relaxed cat may tolerate much that is unacceptable about the litter box, whereas a stressed cat may have a lower threshold for substandard toileting conditions.[14] Addressing environmental and social stress is therefore an essential part of treating litter box aversions.

For cats with a substrate preference, the appropriate toileting area should be optimized as described elsewhere in this article. The inappropriate substrate should be made less attractive and/or unavailable. For example, targeted throw rugs can be removed and doors to targeted bedrooms can be closed. Upside-down cleated rug runners can be placed on furniture to make it less attractive. If the underlying cause of the problem is not addressed, a cat may find other unacceptable places to eliminate when denied access to the preferred substrate.[8,10] For cats with a location preference, a litter box can be placed in the soiled location. Once it is used consistently, it can be gradually relocated at a rate of 1 inch per day to a more acceptable area for the owner.[17] Although some authors recommend changing the function of the soiled area by placing a food bowl in that location, others do not.[8,16]

Confinement has been recommended to treat cats with aversions and preferences. The cat is placed in a large cage or small room with a litter box and then gradually allowed more freedom when he starts using the box.[21] It may be necessary to limit a cat's movement by preventing access to areas that are difficult to clean while the problem is being solved, but extended confinement is likely to cause an increase in anxiety and stress.[43] If a cat must be confined to prevent further property damage, attention should be given to the cat's need for environmental enrichment and social engagement.[18]

Owners must be counseled not to reprimand or punish their cat when urine is found outside of the litter box. For a cat to make an association between the behavior and the consequence, a punishment must be delivered within 1 second of the unwanted behavior. Random delayed scolding or punishment is likely to increase his anxiety and thus increase inappropriate toileting. Some authors recommend interrupting the cat when he is caught in the act of urinating outside the box by startling the cat from a distance so that the cat does not make a negative association with the owner.[21] Punishing or even startling a cat when caught eliminating risks adding to the problem by increasing anxiety and fear.[8,14,16] Herron[18] recommends an interrupter cue that may stop a cat from urinating without causing fear. To create the cue, a neutral sound such as a bell or crinkling sound of a treat bag is associated with a food treat by classical conditioning. When the cat shows signs of preparing to eliminate outside the box, the cue is given to interrupt the behavior and the cat is rewarded. The cat is then taken to the box and given another treat if he eliminates.[18]

Although most studies focus on the use of pheromone therapy for the treatment of marking, pheromones may be helpful for treating nonmarking inappropriate elimination if there is evidence of anxiety.[18] Psychoactive medication is rarely beneficial for the treatment of litter box aversion or substrate preference, except when avoidance of the box is motivated by anxiety or fear.[8,10,14] In this author's clinical experience, a 12-week course of buspirone was helpful in treating a cat with learned fear of the litter box after an episode of obstipation.

CANINE INAPPROPRIATE ELIMINATION
Normal Canine Elimination

The ability to housetrain dogs is predicated on their instinct not to soil the nesting area. Between 2 and 3 weeks of age, puppies begin to move away from the nest to eliminate.[44] At 5 weeks of age, puppies begin to eliminate in a defined area.[45] Careful avoidance of unwanted elimination and rewarding of appropriate behavior supports the development of house training through classical and operant conditioning.[45]

Diagnosing Inappropriate Elimination

As with cats, the key to effective treatment for canine periuria is a correct diagnosis arrived at by systematic approach.

Is it medical or behavioral?

Before a behavioral diagnosis is made, medical causes of periuria should be ruled out with a physical examination and basic database that includes a complete blood count, chemistry panel, urinalysis, and urine culture. Depending on the physical examination findings and laboratory results, additional testing and/or imaging may be warranted. Urinary tract disease, kidney disease, pyometra, and metabolic disorders such as diabetes mellitus, diabetes insipidus, and Cushing's disease may cause pollakiuria, dysuria, or polyuria that results in house soiling. Iatrogenic causes such as medication that increases urination should be considered. Medications such as prednisone may cause polyuria. Gonadectomized females are at an increased risk of incontinence secondary to sphincter incompetence. Diseases that limit mobility such as osteoarthritis or hip dysplasia may make it difficult to descend stairs to the outside.[45,46] For older dogs, cognitive dysfunction must be considered. Loss of house training is one of the central clinical signs of canine cognitive dysfunction. Other signs are loss of recognition and cognition, disorientation, and changes in the sleep–wake cycle. There are no perimortem tests for cognitive dysfunction. It is a diagnosis of exclusion made on the basis of history and clinical observation.[47]

A Detailed History

The history should include information about the volume, location, substrate, and timing of the patient's accidents; whether the patient urinates in front of the owner; and the owner's response when finding urine. The frequency of elimination opportunities, whether the owner is present with the dog when he urinates, and how the owner responds are also relevant. Background information about the patient's household the presence of children and other animals should be collected. Information about other behavior problems should be included as well, such as noise phobia, fear of conspecifics, and interdog housemate aggression. Changes in the environment or schedule such as new canine neighbors or visitors, or a recent stay at a boarding kennel should be noted.

Diagnostic Categories for Behavioral Periuria

The primary diagnostic categories for canine urination problems are insufficient or lapsed house training, urine marking, anxiety and fear-based urination, submissive and excitement urination, and improper management.

Management Issues

House soiling may be the result of unrealistic expectations. Owners may not appreciate how frequently dogs need to relieve themselves, especially when very young or very old. Puppies can be expected to wait 1 hour plus 1 to 2 hours for each month of life between eliminations, depending on the size of the dog.[48] Healthy adult dogs can be expected to hold their urine for 6 hours.[46] A lack of careful management may also be the problem. For example, dogs that are not supervised when let out to urinate may become distracted, come in before urinating, and urinate later in the house. Dogs that are brought in immediately after eliminating may learn to hold their urine to remain outside longer. If they are brought in without urinating, they may go inside at a later time.[45]

Treatment for Management Problems

Owner education about appropriate management and realistic, age-appropriate expectations is the best treatment.

Fear and anxiety

Inappropriate elimination is a commonly reported clinical sign of separation anxiety, along with destructiveness and vocalization.[49] Dogs with separation anxiety only display clinical signs in the absence of the owner. Dogs with phobias, such as thunderstorm phobia, may eliminate when exposed to the frightening stimuli. In addition to urination that occurs in direct response to fear or startle, dogs may develop a persistent fear of the area where they encountered the frightening stimulus. For example, if she heard a loud crack of thunder in the yard, she may avoid the yard long after the storm has passed. Patients with a history of severe punishment when urinating indoors in front of their owners may wait to eliminate when they are left alone in the house, safely away from the owner.

Effective resolution of fear-based elimination issues depends on treating the underlying causes, such as separation distress and noise phobia with environmental management, behavior modification, and antianxiety medication if indicated.

Incomplete or lapsed house training

Dogs with incomplete or lost house training produce a volume of urine that is consistent with emptying of the bladder. The frequency is identical to that of a normal dog. A patient may eliminate indoors and outdoors, and in the presence and/or the absence of the owner depending on when she has the urge. Urine deposits are not associated with locations that have territorial or social significance, and they do not occur in association with signs of fear. Some patients with incomplete training may seek out areas of the home that are rarely used and may thus be considered outside of the dog's core living space. Dogs with a history of being forced to eliminate when confined may lose the natural tendency to eliminate away from the core living area. Dogs that have always lived outside do not learn to distinguish between indoors and outdoors when urinating.[46] Some dogs will urinate when their owners are away too often. It is insecurity, not retribution.

Incomplete or lapsed house training is addressed by repeating puppy house training. During remedial training, the dog should be taken on a leash to urinate in a designated outdoor location at regular intervals. Dogs usually eliminate during transitions between activities, for example, after awakening, eating, or playing, and before going to bed. When first starting, the dog may need to go out once every hour. When he is taken to his elimination spot, he should be walked around until he urinates. When he has emptied his bladder, the owner should immediately praise him lavishly, give him a food treat, and then allow him to play and explore. Timing is everything. Praise and rewards must be given immediately after the dog urinates. Giving the treat when he comes inside teaches him that returning to the house, not urinating outside, is the desired behavior.[45,46,48] If the dog does not urinate within several minutes, he should be brought back inside and confined to prevent an accident. A crate without absorbent bedding will work well for dogs that are already crate trained. The umbilical cord method is preferable for dogs that are not accustomed to crating. The dog is tethered to the owner on a short leash. He is unlikely to urinate on a short leash because he cannot move away when he has finished. Also, the proximity of the owner enables him to observe preeliminatory behaviors such as circling, sniffing, or vocalizing, and immediately take the dog out.

To prevent dogs from being attracted back to soiled areas in the house, all urine must be thoroughly cleaned and treated with odor-mitigating products. Block the dog's access to areas that cannot be thoroughly rid of residual urine smell.

Delayed punishment for inappropriate elimination is counterproductive. Dogs do not associate the previous act of soiling with punishment or scolding that takes place well after the act. The guilty look that owners report when finding a puddle of urine reflects the dog's fear and attempt to placate the incomprehensibly angry owner. Even when caught in flagrante delicto, harsh punishment is more likely to cause a fear of eliminating in front of the owner or even fear of the owner. A gentle interruption, such as clapping and calling his name, followed by a trip outside where he can be praised and rewarded for completing his business, will be more effective.

Overall Marking

Marking is a normal canine behavior that functions to communicate information about sexual status, social threat, and territorial boundaries.[50] It is a sexually dimorphic behavior that occurs in males with greater frequency. Females are more likely to mark during estrus. Both intact and neutered males mark in the presence of a female in estrus. The presence of nonresident dogs in or near a dog's home may trigger inappropriate marking.[45] In free-roaming dogs, urine marks correspond with areas where dogs outside of the social group are encountered, which suggests territorial defense.[51] Dogs also mark novel objects such as packages, luggage, or new furniture brought into the home. In a study of free-roaming dogs in India, dogs marked unfamiliar vehicles that parked in their territory. Researchers have speculated that dogs may mark novel objects to make them more familiar and thus less concerning.[51]

As with cats, canine urine marking may also be stimulated by stress in both sexes, regardless of neuter status.[46,52] Social stress such as agonistic interactions with other animals in the home and environmental stress such as insufficient exercise or isolation may stimulate urine marking. Dogs that mark inside generally go outside to empty their bladders. Because urine marking is about communication, dogs mark significant places and objects such as doors and windows, or items associated with household members. The volume of urine deposited by marking is small.[45,48]

Urine Marking

Eliminating the triggers best treats marking. For dogs motivated by territoriality, it is best to avoid having other dogs visit the home. Also, neighborhood dogs should be discouraged from marking near the house. Pull the shades if the dog marks next to the windows. Keep new items picked up or blocked off until the dog has had an opportunity to become familiar with the object.[45] Triggers of anxious marking such as social problems between canine housemates must be identified and treated.

Neutering may be helpful. However, the benefits are much less pronounced in dogs than in cats. In a retrospective cohort study of 57 male dogs, castration resulted in a 50% or greater improvement in 60% of dogs, and 90% improvement in 25% to 40% of dogs.[53] In a prospective study of 7 male dogs, no change in marking behavior was noticed 5 months after castration.[54]

Whereas there is a wealth of research about pharmacologic treatments for feline urine marking, there is a dearth of research about canine urine marking. Nevertheless, psychoactive medication can be effective at reducing urine marking by raising the threshold for anxiety and reactivity.[45,46] In this author's clinical experience, selective serotonin reuptake inhibitors (fluoxetine, sertraline, and paroxetine) or tricyclic antidepressants (clomipramine) may be a beneficial addition to the treatment plan. Adverse effects of selective serotonin reuptake inhibitors include lethargy, decreased appetite, gastrointestinal disturbance, hyponatremia, and agitation.[55] Clomipramine may cause sedation, appetite changes, regurgitation, and anticholinergic effects.[56] The anticholinergic effect of urine retention may be beneficial when treating urine marking.[57]

Submissive Urination

Submissive urination is most common in young female dogs that are otherwise house trained. Gestures that a dog perceives as frightening such as approaching, reaching over, petting, speaking loudly, staring, and punishment or scolding trigger the release of urine.[48] Submissive urination is accompanied by other signs of fear and social deference such as a lowered body posture, horizontally retracted lips, or lateral recumbency with a leg elevated.[45,46]

Changing the way in which owners interact with their dog is usually effective. Owners should remain calm when greeting the dog and allow her to approach when she is ready. Leaning over or reaching toward her should be avoided. Teaching alternative, nonsubmissive behaviors, such as sitting on cue for a food reward when greeting, reduces anxiety by making the interaction predictable.[58] Owners must be informed that punishment or scolding will intensify the problem. Pharmacologic therapy such a tricyclic antidepressant, selective serotonin reuptake inhibitor, or buspirone may also be added to treat the patient's anxiety. Submissive urination frequently resolves with age.

Excitement Urination

Dogs diagnosed with excitement urination evacuate their bladders when aroused or excited. They usually do not squat or lift a leg and often seem unaware that the bladder has been released. Excitement urination is most common in young dogs that lack neuromuscular control when excited.[46]

Like submissive urination, excitement urination is a problem of young dogs that generally resolves with age. To facilitate resolution of the problem, owners should avoid getting the dog overly excited. A dog can be taught to self-calm by rewarding relaxed and settled behavior or teaching him to settle into a relaxed down on cue.

OWNER EDUCATION

An important barrier to successful resolution of the canine and feline house soiling is the misconception that owners have about inappropriate urination. Clients frequently believe that cats and dogs urinate in the home out of vindictiveness.[46] Owner education must be a part of the treatment plan. If owners understand that their pet is not angry or spiteful, they may be more motivated to pursue treatment rather than relinquishment.

PROGNOSIS

The prognosis for inappropriate urination for cats and dogs is good if there are no medical comorbidities.[8] In 1 study, 84% of the cases presented for inappropriate elimination at Cornell University Animal Behavior Clinic resolved.[59]

REFERENCES

1. Scarlett JM, Salman MD, New JG, et al. The role of veterinary practitioners in reducing dog and cat relinquishments and euthanasias. J Am Vet Med Assoc 2002;220(3):306–11.
2. Patronek GJ, Glickman LT, Beck AM, et al. Risk factors for relinquishment of cats to an animal shelter. J Am Vet Med Assoc 1996;209(3):582–8.
3. Patronek GJ, Glickman LT, Beck AM, et al. Risk factors for relinquishment of dogs to an animal shelter. J Am Vet Med Assoc 1996;209(3):572–81.
4. Knesl O, Hart BL, Fine AH, et al. Opportunities for incorporating the human-animal bond in companion animal practice. J Am Vet Med Assoc 2016;249(1): 42–4.
5. Calder CD, Albright JD, Koch C. Evaluating graduating veterinary students' perception of preparedness in clinical veterinary behavior for "Day 1" practice and the factors which influence that perception: a questionnaire-based survey. J Vet Behav 2017;20:116–20.
6. Bergman L, Hart BL, Bain M, et al. Evaluation of urine marking by cats as a model for understanding veterinary diagnostic and treatment approaches and client attitudes. J Am Vet Med Assoc 2002;221(9):1282–6.
7. Lilly LM. Evaluation of behavior knowledge in first year veterinary students before and after an introduction to behavior course. In: ACVB Behavior Symposium Proceedings. July 12, 2018, Denver, CO.
8. Dantas LMS. Vertical or horizontal? Diagnosing and treating cats who urinate outside the box. Vet Clin Small Anim 2018;48:03–417.
9. Barcelos AM, McPeake K, Affenzeller N, et al. Common risk factors for urinary house soiling (Periuria) in cats and its differentiation: the sensitivity and specificity of common diagnostic signs. Front Vet Sci 2018;5:108.
10. Neilson J. Thinking outside the box: feline elimination. J Feline Med Surg 2004;6: 5–11.
11. Overall KL. Feline elimination disorders. Undesirable, problematic and abnormal feline behavior and behavioral pathologies. In: Manual of clinical behavioral medicine for dogs and cats. St Louis (MO): Elsevier; 2013. p. 360–457.
12. Beaver BV. Feline eliminative behavior. In: Beaver BV, editor. Feline behavior: a guide for veterinarians. 2nd edition. St Louis (MO): Saunders; 2003. p. 247–73.
13. Olm DD, Houpt KA. Feline house-soiling problems. J Appl Behav Sci 1988;20(3): 335–45.
14. Neilson J. House soiling by cats. In: Horwitz DF, Mills DS, editors. BSAVA manual of canine and feline behavioural medicine. 2nd edition. Gloucester (England): BSAVA; 2009. p. 98–110.
15. Landsberg GM, Malamed R. Clinical picture of canine and feline cognitive impairment. In: Landsberg G, Mad'ari A, Žilka N, editors. Canine and feline dementia

molecular basis, diagnostics and therapy. Cham (Switzerland): Springer International Publishing AG; 2017. p. 1–12.

16. Carney HC, Sadek TP, Curtis TM, et al. AAFP and ISFM guidelines for diagnosing and solving house-soiling behavior in cats. J Feline Med Surg 2014;16:579–98.

17. Neilson JC. Feline house soiling: elimination and marking behaviors. Vet Clin North Am Small Anim Pract 2003;33(2):287–301.

18. Herron ME. Advances in understanding and treatment of feline inappropriate elimination. Top Companion Anim Med 2010;25(4):195–202.

19. Buffington CA, Chew DJ, Woodworth BE. Feline interstitial cystitis. J Am Vet Med Assoc 1999;215(5):682–7.

20. Gunn-Moore DA. Cognitive dysfunction in cats: clinical assessment and management. Top Companion Anim Med 2011;26(1):17–24.

21. Landsberg G, Hunthausen W, Ackerman L. Feline housesoiling. In: Landsberg G, Hunthausen W, Ackerman L, editors. Handbook of behavior problems of the dog and cat. 2nd edition. Edinburgh (Scotland): Saunders; 2003. p. 365–84.

22. Schwartz S. Separation anxiety syndrome in cats: 136 cases (1991-2000). J Am Vet Med Assoc 2002;220(7):1028–33.

23. Hart BL, Barrett RE. Effects of castration on fighting, roaming, and urine spraying in adult male cats. J Am Vet Med Assoc 1973;163(3):290–2.

24. Ellis SL, Rodan I, Carney HC, et al. AAFP and ISFM feline environmental needs guideline. J Feline Med Surg 2013;15:219–30.

25. Pryor PA, Hart BL, Bain MJ, et al. Causes of urine marking in cats and effects of environmental management on frequency of marking. J Am Vet Med Assoc 2001; 219(12):1709–13.

26. Pageat P, Gaultier E. Current research in canine and feline pheromones. Vet Clin North Am Small Anim Pract 2003;33(2):187–211.

27. Mills D, Redgate SE, Landsberg GM. A meta-analysis of treatments for feline urine spraying. PLoS One 2011;6(4):1–9.

28. Hunthausen W. Evaluating a feline facial pheromone analogue to control urine spraying. Vet Med 2000;95:151–6.

29. Pryor PA, Hart BL, Cliff KD, et al. Effects of a selective serotonin reuptake inhibitor on urine spraying behavior in cats. J Am Vet Med Assoc 2001;219(11):1557–61.

30. Landsberg GM, Wilson AL. Effects of clomipramine on cats presented for urine marking. J Am Vet Med Assoc 2005;41(1):3–11.

31. King JN, Steffan J, Heath SE, et al. Determination of the dosage of clomipramine for the treatment of urine spraying in cats. J Am Vet Med Assoc 2004;225(6): 881–7.

32. Hart BL, Eckstein RA, Powell KL, et al. Effectiveness of buspirone on urine spraying and inappropriate urination in cats. J Am Vet Med Assoc 1993;203(2):254–8.

33. Cooper L, Hart BL. Comparison of diazepam with progestin for effectiveness in suppression of urine spraying behavior in cats. J Am Vet Med Assoc 1992; 200(6):797–801.

34. Hughes D, Moreau RE, Overall KL, et al. Acute hepatic necrosis and liver failure associated with benzodiazepine therapy in six cats, 1986-1995. J Vet Emerg Crit Car 1996;6(1):13–20.

35. Sung W, Crowell-Davis SL. Elimination behavior patterns of domestic cats (Felis catus) with and without elimination behavior problems. Am J Vet Res 2006; 67(9):1500–4.

36. Ellis JJ, McGowan RTS, Martin F. Does previous use affect litter box appeal in multi-cat households? Behav Processes 2017;141(Pt 3):284–90.

37. Beaver BV, Terry ML, LaSagna CL, et al. Effectiveness of products in eliminating cat urine odors from carpet. J Am Vet Med Assoc 1989;194(11):1589–91.
38. Cottam N, Dodman NH. Effect of an odor eliminator on feline litter box behavior. J Feline Med Surg 2007;9(1):44–50.
39. Grigg EK, Pick L, Nibblett B. Litter box preference in domestic cats: covered versus uncovered. J Feline Med Surg 2013;15(4):280–4.
40. Guy NC, Hopson M, Vanderstichel R. Litterbox size preference in domestic cats (Felis catus). J Vet Behav 2014;9(2):78–82.
41. Horwitz DF. Behavioral and environmental factors associated with elimination behavior problems in cats: a retrospective study. Appl Anim Behav Sci 1997; 52:129–37.
42. Borchelt PL. Cat elimination behavior problems. Vet Clin North Am Small Anim Pract 1991;21(2):257–64.
43. Horwitz DF, Neilson JC. House soiling: feline. In: Blackwell's five-minute veterinary consult clinical companion. Ames (IA): Blackwell; 2007. p. 329–36.
44. Serpell J, Duffy DL, Jagoe JA. Becoming a dog: early experience and the development of behavior. In: Serpell J, editor. The domestic dog its evolution, behavior and interactions with people. 2nd edition. Cambridge (England): Cambridge University Press; 2017. p. 93–117.
45. Landsberg G, Hunthausen W, Ackerman L. Canine housesoiling. In: Landsberg G, Hunthausen W, Ackerman L, editors. Handbook of behavior problems of the dog and cat. 2nd edition. Edinburgh (Scotland): Saunders; 2003. p. 349–64.
46. Overall KL. Feline elimination disorders. Abnormal canine behaviors and behavioral pathologies not primarily involving pathological aggression. In: Manual of clinical behavioral medicine for dogs and cats. St Louis (MO): Elsevier; 2013. p. 231–311.
47. Frank D. Cognitive dysfunction in dogs. In: Hill's European Symposium on Canine Brain Ageing. Barcelona, Spain, 2002. Available at: https://www.ivis.org/proceedings/hills/brain/toc.asp. Accessed August 1, 2018.
48. Houpt KA. House soiling by dogs. In: Horwitz DF, Mills DS, editors. BSAVA manual of canine and feline behavioural medicine. 2nd edition. Gloucester (England): BSAVA; 2009. p. 111–6.
49. Landsberg GM, Melese P, Sherman BL, et al. Effectiveness of fluoxetine chewable tablets in the treatment of canine separation anxiety. J Vet Behav 2008; 3(1):12–9.
50. Cafazzo S, Natoli E, Valsecchi P. Scent marking behaviour in a pack of free ranging domestic dogs. Ethology 2012;118:1–12.
51. Pal SK. Urine marking by free-ranging dogs (Canis familiaris) in relation to sex, season, place and posture. Appl Anim Behav Sci 2003;80:45–59.
52. Lindell E. Canine house soiling. Clinicians brief. 2017. Available at: https://files.brief.vet/migration/article/35531/ab_canine-house-soiling-35531-article.pdf. Accessed September 3, 2018.
53. Neilson JC, Eckstein RA, Hart BL. Effects of castration on problem behaviors in male dogs with reference to age and duration of behavior. J Am Vet Med Assoc 1997;211(2):180–2.
54. Hart BL. Environmental and hormonal influences on urine marking behavior in the adult dog. Behav Biol 1974;11(2):167–76.
55. Crowell-Davis S, Murray T. Selective serotonin reuptake inhibitors. In: Veterinary psychopharmacology. Oxford (England): Blackwell Publishing; 2006. p. 80–110.

56. Crowell-Davis S, Murray T. Tricyclic antidepressants. In: Veterinary psychophar-macology. Oxford (England): Blackwell Publishing; 2006. p. 179–206.
57. King JN, Simpson BS, Overall KL, et al. Treatment of separation anxiety in dogs with clomipramine: results from a prospective, randomized, double-blind, pla-cebo-controlled, parallel-group, multicenter clinical trial. Appl Anim Behav Sci 2000;67(4):255–75.
58. Pryor P. Animal behavior case of the month. J Am Vet Med Assoc 2003;223(6): 790–2.
59. Yeon SC, Erb HN, Houpt KA. A retrospective study of canine house soiling: diag-nosis and treatment. J Am Anim Hosp Assoc 1999;35(2):101–6.

Medical and Interventional Management of Upper Urinary Tract Uroliths

Melissa Milligan, vmd*, Allyson C. Berent, dvm

KEYWORDS

- Endoscopic nephrolithotomy • Endourology
- Extracorporeal shockwave lithotripsy (ESWL) • Nephrolithiasis • Stone dissolution
- Subcutaneous ureteral bypass device (SUB) • Ureteral obstruction
- Ureteral stenting

KEY POINTS

1. Nephroliths are often clinically silent. When non-obstructive and of an amenable stone type, dissolution should be attempted.
2. When problematic, nephrolithotomy can be considered. Depending on stone type, size, and species, extracorporeal shockwave lithotripsy or endoscopic nephrolithotomy are preferred techniques.
3. Obstructive ureterolithiasis should be addressed immediately to preserve kidney function. Because of decreased morbidity and mortality and versatility for all causes, interventional techniques for kidney decompression are preferred by the authors.
4. Proper training and expertise in these interventional techniques should be acquired before performing them on clinical patients for the best possible outcomes.

INTRODUCTION

Upper urinary tract uroliths are a common problem in our small animal patients and are being more commonly recognized with the increased use of diagnostic imaging as part of a minimum database. Appropriate medical, surgical, and/or interventional management is necessary for the best outcomes and preservation of kidney function. In many instances, canine and feline nephroliths are clinically silent for many years, whereas ureteroliths are typically found as a more urgent clinical dilemma. However, when nephroliths are problematic, or become obstructive ureteroliths, intervention is

Disclosure Statement: Dr A.C. Berent is a consultant for Norfolk Vet Products and Infiniti Medical, LLC, both of which distribute various medical devices that are discussed in this article. Dr M. Milligan has nothing to disclose.
The Animal Medical Center, 510 East 62nd Street, New York, NY 10065, USA
* Corresponding author.
E-mail address: Melissa.Milligan@amcny.org

Vet Clin Small Anim 49 (2019) 157–174
https://doi.org/10.1016/j.cvsm.2018.11.004

vetsmall.theclinics.com

indicated. The content of this article is based on best evidence, when available, although much is the anecdotal experience of the authors.

NEPHROLITHIASIS

Most nephroliths found in canine and feline patients are clinically silent for many years and require diligent monitoring to ensure they do not mobilize to become a ureteral outflow tract obstruction. Dissolution of upper urinary tract stones should always be attempted when non-obstructive and stone type is amenable (eg, struvite, +/− urate and cysteine). The best practice to accomplish stone dissolution is described in the sections below.

MEDICAL MANAGEMENT

Dissolution of upper urinary tract stones should always be attempted when non-obstructive and stone type is amenable, and given the likelihood of stone recurrence in many cases, preventative measures should be instituted whenever possible. Stone type can often be carefully predicted when considering signalment, radiographic appearance, urine microbiologic culture, fasted and fresh urine pH, fresh urine crystals, or, when available qualitative and quantitative crystallographic analysis. We use these predictions to help make decisions on the best treatment options for the patient (**Table 1**).

Struvite Dissolution and Prevention

Canine upper tract uroliths have been reported to be of struvite content in 50% to 60% of cases.[1–3] Feline upper tract stones, on the other hand, are rarely composed of struvite, with 92% being calcium oxalate and 8% being dried solidified blood stones.[3,4] Struvite uroliths are composed of magnesium ammonium phosphate hexahydrate, and are more likely to form when urine is oversaturated with these minerals. In canine patients, struvite uroliths typically occur secondary to a urinary tract infection that is associated with urease-producing bacteria, such as *Staphylococcus* spp, *Proteus* spp, or *Klebsiella* spp. Bacterial urease converts urea to ammonia thus making the urine alkaline. This increase in urine pH results in precipitation of calcium and magnesium phosphates, and subsequent aggregation and stone formation. Female dogs are more likely than male dogs to be affected with struvite stones owing to their increased risk for ascending urinary tract infections.[1,3] This is likely secondary to their shorter and wider urethra, and the close association of the vulva to the anus. Struvite uroliths classically have a radiopaque appearance, are a rounded shape with some flat surfaces, and can be excessively large at times (**Fig. 1**). In the kidney, these stones are often a staghorn appearance, forming the shape of the renal pelvis and protruding into the calices and down the proximal ureter (see **Fig. 1**).

Sterile struvite stones have been reported, but are rare in dogs.[5] In cats, however, sterile struvite stones are more typical, so dissolution does not typically require antibiotics.[6] However, struvite stones in cats are typically only found in the lower urinary tract. If stones are visualized in the kidneys or ureters on radiograph in a cat than they are nearly always calcium oxalate in composition.[7]

Struvite stones can typically be dissolved in essentially all cases, regardless of their size, number, or location, as long as they are non-obstructive, surrounded by urine, and composed of purely magnesium ammonium and phosphate, rather than mixed with calcium apatite/phosphate. In the event a struvite stone is causing a ureteral obstruction than a stent would be ideal to decompress the collection system and allow urine to drain around the stone while dissolution occurs. Dissolution of ureteroliths

Table 1
Upper tract stone type predictions

	Signalment	Sex and Species	pH (Fasting and Fresh)	Crystals	Radiographic Appearance	Presence of Infection
Struvite	Any breed	Female canines	>7.0	Variable/ unpredictable	Staghorn/soft/rounded	Present: urease-producing bacteria
Urate	Dalmatians, Bulldogs, PSS dogs, or cat	Canine > feline, male or female	<7.0	Usually present	Minimally opaque, staghorn	Absent
Cystine	English Bulldogs, Newfoundlands, Mastiffs, Labrador Retrievers, male intact dogs	Canine, male and female	Variable	Usually present	Large, minimally opaque	Absent
Calcium oxalate	Terriers, Schnauzers, Shih Tzu, Poodles, other metabolic derangement for hypercalciuria	Canines and feline, male and female	<7.0	Variable/ unpredictable	Very opaque, sharp and irregular, small or large, mix mineralization	Absent

Abbreviation: PSS, **portosystemic shunt.**

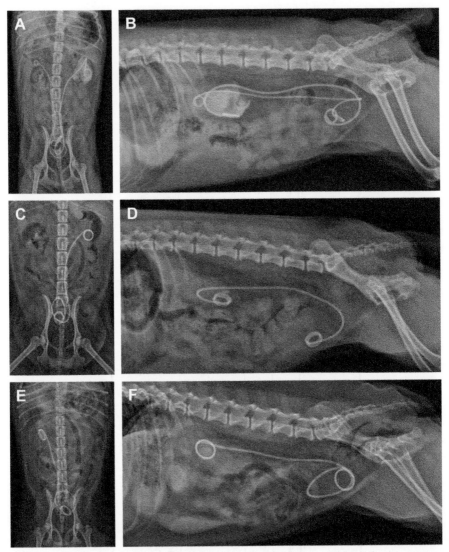

Fig. 1. Radiographs of dogs with renoliths of varying stone types. (*A*) Mixed calcium stone. Note the staghorn appearance in the ventrodorsal view. (*B*) Struvite renoliths. (*C, D*) Cystine renoliths. Note the oval shape. (*E, F*) Calcium oxalate renoliths. Note the sharp and irregular outline, and relative radiopacity.

often takes 2 to 6 weeks. Appropriate dissolution management involves instituting appropriate antibiotic therapy beyond the entire course of stone resolution, and promoting an acidic urine pH either with medication (eg, DL-methionine: 75–100 mg/kg po q12) or a neutral urine pH that is controlled through a diet where the key minerals of the stone are limited (eg, Hill's C/D or Royal Canine Urinary SO).[1,3,8] Care should be taken to avoid acidification if stone type is unknown and the clinician is performing a dissolution trial without clear evidence of struvite composition. In that case neutral urine pH with a dissolution diet, while controlling the urinary tract infection, is the safest approach. Inappropriate acidification could result in progression of calcium oxalate stone size and number. Increased water intake should be encouraged to achieve a urine-specific gravity of less than 1.020. Owners should add 1 to 2 additional walks per day to encourage bladder and crystal elimination.

Although stone dissolution is being implemented, repeat urinalysis (with a fasted urine pH), urine culture, and radiographs are serially recommended every 4 weeks. This is to monitor dissolution progress. In the authors' experience, within 2 to 6 weeks ureteroliths should be nearly dissolved, and within 3 months nephroliths should have decreased in size by greater than 25%. Time to full dissolution can take 6 to 9 months for large nephroliths, and the authors recommend that antibiotic therapy should be continued at the full dose for 4 weeks beyond when the stones are radiographically absent. Bacteria can be gradually released from the stone matrix as dissolution occurs, and maintaining antibiotic treatment is mandatory to ensure that additional struvite deposition does not occur.[9] Following complete dissolution, routine serial urine testing is recommended to monitor and treat infections as early as possible. They are often recurrent infections, but prompt treatment will prevent future stone formation. If, despite appropriate treatment and owner compliance, the stone is not dissolving, than stone removal should be considered. Consideration should be given to addressing any anatomic or functional risk factors for recurrent urinary tract infections (eg, recessed vulva, persistent paramesonephric remnant, urinary incontinence, urachal diverticulum).

Urate Dissolution and Prevention

Urate stones include stones composed of uric acid, ammonium urate, ammonium biurate, and other salts of uric acid. Factors that promote urate urolith formation include hyperuricosuria, concentrated urine, and an acidic pH. In normal cats and dogs, uric acid is formed as an intermediate product of purine metabolism in the liver. Purines are converted to hypoxanthine, then to xanthine, and then to uric acid by xanthine oxidase. Uric acid is then converted to allantoin by uricase. Allantoin is highly water soluble and is excreted in urine. Thus, dogs with portovascular anomalies, or defects in uric acid transport, are predisposed to urate stone formation. Mutations in the LC2A9 gene that encodes for urate transport in the liver and kidney has been identified Dalmatians, English Bulldogs, and Black Russian Terriers.[10–12] This genetic disorder follows an autosomal recessive pattern of inheritance. The mutation results in decreased conversion of uric acid to allantoin and hyperuricasemia. There is no re-absorption of uric acid following glomerular filtration, and thus hyperuricuria, which results in stone formation.

In cats with urate stones, the pathogenesis is less clear. One theory is that, being strict carnivores, cats have limited ability to upregulate and downregulate the production of catabolic enzymes of amino acid metabolism. Thus, increased dietary protein results in increased purine formation and oversaturation of urea in the urine. Portovascular anomalies in cats, as well as dogs, can also result in stone formation.[13] Urate stones are typically radiolucent but can be visible, minimally so, on radiographs. Dogs with urate stones most commonly have urate crystalluria on a fresh urine sample.

Urate stones are amenable to medical dissolution. However, medical dissolution is only considered effective approximately 30% of the time.[14] In the face of uncorrected liver disease, dissolution is not considered medically appropriate, as the medications target xanthine oxidase in the liver, and cannot be appropriately metabolized. Care should be taken to appropriately screen patients for portovascular anomalies with serum bile acid testing, protein C levels and/or diagnostic imaging. For dissolution, a purine-restricted diet that promotes an alkaline urine pH should be fed exclusively.[14–16] Allopurinol, a xanthine oxidase inhibitor, can be given at a dose of 15 mg/kg po q12 to inhibit conversion of xanthine to uric acid.[16] However, care should be taken as this medication can promote xanthine stone formation if purine intake is not controlled.[17] If, despite appropriate medical management, dissolution is not achieved, removal of problematic stones should be considered.

Cystine Dissolution and Prevention

Cystine uroliths are composed of cystine molecules linked by disulfide bonds, and occur with hyperexcretion of cystine in urine.[18] Cystine stones can be suspected when there are multiple small ovoid stones with minimal radiopacity (see **Table1**). Because of the small size and minimal radiopacity, ultrasound can be a helpful diagnostic tool for detection. Cystine crystals are commonly seen in the fresh urine sample of dogs with cystine stones and should be carefully assessed. Cystine stones are more commonly found in dogs than cats, and in male dogs over females.[19] Overrepresented breeds include Newfoundlands, Mastiffs, English Bulldogs, Labrador Retrievers, Irish Terriers, Scottish Deerhounds, Corgis, Australian Cattle Dogs, and Chihuahuas.[19]

In normal urine filtration, the cystine amino acid passes through the glomerular filtration barrier and is reabsorbed in the proximal convoluted tubule. In patients with cystinuria, there is a defect in the carrier proteins responsible for re-absorption of cystine. This defect can be the result of a mutation in a gene that affects appropriate function of these receptors in the proximal convoluted tubule, such as the SLC3A1 or the SLC7A9 gene.[20] The mutation in the SLC3A1 is at exon 2 and encodes for a renal basic amino acid transporter. This is the most common mutation in Labrador Retrievers.[20] The mutation in the SLC7A9 gene encodes intramembrane transporter protein, and this is most commonly found in Miniature pinchers.[20] Genetic screening is available for the recognized mutations and for testosterone-associated cystinuria. Testosterone-associated cystinuria has been reported in Mastiffs, Scottish Deerhounds, and Irish Terriers, and neutering is the recommended treatment.[21]

For the dissolution of cystine stones, a restricted-amino acid diet that is low in cystine, while also promoting alkaline urine pH (>7.5), should be fed exclusively. In addition chelators such as 2-mercaptopropionylglycine (20 mg/kg po q12 h) could be considered, and are reported to be effective in dissolving stones in approximately 53% of cases.[22] The addition of potassium citrate can also be considered. Neutering has been associated with decreased cystinuria in specific breeds of dogs.[20] If dissolution is not successful, or the cost of the medication is prohibitive, than removal of the stones can be considered, when necessary.

Calcium Oxalate Prevention

Calcium oxalate stones are the most common stone type in both dogs and cats, and are most likely to form with hypercalciuria.[23–25] Hypercalciuria can occur secondary to various pathologic processes including: increased jejunal absorption of calcium, impaired renal tubular re-absorption of calcium, increased bone demineralization, metabolic acidosis, primary hyperparathyroidism, and feline idiopathic hypercalcemia. Hypercalciuria can occur with certain medications and dietary factors including loop diuretics, corticosteroids, urinary acidifiers, increased dietary calcium, increased intake of vitamins C and D, and low B6.[26–28] Hyperoxaluria has been reported to occur in dogs in which there is decreased degradation of dietary oxalate secondary to decreased enteric *Oxalobacter formigenes*.[29]

Male dogs are over-represented for developing calcium oxalate stones, as are several breeds including Bichon Frise, Cairn Terriers, Chihuahuas, Lhasa Apso, Pomeranians,

Maltese, Miniature Schnauzers, Shih Tzu, Keeshond, Yorkshire Terriers, Mini Poodles, and Chihuahuas. Calcium oxalate stones can be suspected when radiographs show uroliths that are moderately to markedly radiopaque with sharp projections, and in feline patients in which there are radiopaque upper tract stones (nephroliths and/or ureteroliths) (**Fig. 2**; see **Table 1**), With calcium oxalate stones the urine pH is usually less than 7.0. A urine culture is most commonly negative, but in some cases secondary urinary tract infections are seen, most typically associated with either *E coli* or *Enterococcus* spp. In addition to imaging and urine testing, total body and ionized calcium levels should be evaluated with parathyroid testing if indicated. Calcium oxalate stones are not amenable to dissolution and therefore require removal or bypass if they are problematic (see treatment options below). However, if they are non-problematic nephroliths or ureteroliths, routine monitoring is recommended.

For prevention of additional stone formation, any known cause of increased calciuria should be addressed. Aiming for a non-acidic urine pH (6.8–7.2) and a specific gravity of less than 1.020 may help in slowing or preventing recurrence. Increased urine concentration also predisposes stone formation, so adding water to food and encouraging drinking is important. Urine-specific gravity should be <1.020 to encourage polyuria and crystal elimination rather than stagnancy. Potassium citrate (50–100 mg/kg po q12) can be given to help prevent aciduria and chelate calcium in the urine.[30] Hydrochlorothiazide (1–2 mg/kg po q12) can also be added.[31,32]

REMOVAL OF PROBLEMATIC NEPHROLITHS

When nephroliths are problematic, removal is warranted. Considerations for nephrolithotomy include: (1) progressive loss of renal parenchyma secondary to increasing stone size, (2) pyelonephritis that is persistent despite appropriate duration of medical management, and (3) obstruction at the ureteropelvic junction with associated of hydronephrosis. Pain associated with nephroliths is usually only present with concurrent obstruction, pyelonephritis, or associated pyonephrosis.

Traditional open surgical options for nephrolithotomy include nephrotomy, pyelotomy, or a salvage ureteronephrectomy. Complications associated with these procedures can result in significant morbidity and mortality.[33–35] One study reports a 10% to

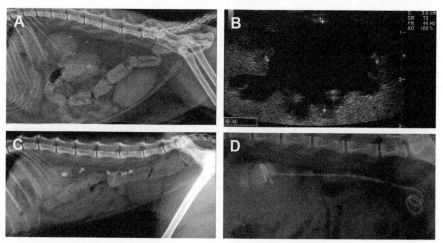

Fig. 2. *A, C)* Cats with multiple calcium oxalate ureteroliths. (*B*) Marked renal pelvic dilation in a cat secondary to obstructive ureterolithiasis. Note the calyx dilation. (*D*) Ureteral stent in a dog placed to relieve an obstruction secondary to multiple calcium oxalate ureteroliths.

20% decrease in glomerular filtration rate when healthy cats underwent a nephrotomy.[34] Nephrotomy would be expected to have a more detrimental effect on kidney function for clinical patients with previous kidney injury and exhaustion of compensatory mechanisms by the time intervention is being pursued. In a report of dogs undergoing traditional surgery for nephrolithiasis, there was a 23% complication rate associated with the procedure and approximately 43% of dogs had some stone fragments remaining after surgery.[35] For the dogs undergoing a nephrectomy, 67% of developed renal azotemia.[35]

Therefore, if stone removal is indicated, decisions on procedures to minimize kidney trauma and preserve kidney function should be considered. The 2016 ACVIM consensus statement on the management of urinary tract stone disease recommends that interventional techniques, such as extracorporeal shockwave lithotripsy (ESWL), percutaneous endoscopic nephrolithotomy, and surgically assisted endoscopic nephrolithotomy, should be considered over traditional surgery to decrease kidney functional loss for stone removal.[36,37]

Extracorporeal Shockwave Lithotripsy

ESWL uses high-energy acoustic pulses to fragment stones into small pieces by creating microcracks in the stone, which expand until fragmentation occurs. The external shockwaves pass through a water medium (water bag), then a coupling gel, through soft tissue structures (eg, skin, muscle, fat, and the kidney/ureter), and then onto the stone(s). Fluoroscopy is typically used to direct the shockwaves onto the stone to ensure the energy is delivered in the appropriate plane. Shock waves of different energy levels are targeted at the stone anywhere from 1000 to 3500 times until fragments are small enough to pass through the ureter and into the urinary bladder for natural voiding.[38,39] However, fragments are typically at least 1 mm in diameter or larger making this technique difficult in very small ureteral lumens, such as the cat (~0.3 mm internal diameter). In addition to the high risk of developing ureteral obstruction, ESWL is not recommended for cats as feline calcium oxalate stones are resistant to fragmentation[21,40] In dogs, treatment is successful, with an 85% success rate and less than 1% mortality rate. However, 30% of dogs require more than one treatment to achieve the necessary degree of fragmentation, and 10% of dogs developed a transient ureteral obstruction as it can take weeks for all of the stone fragments to move into the bladder.[41] This technique is not recommended when the stone diameter is 1.0 to 1.5 cm or greater, as the amount of fragments and debris generated increase the risk for ureteral obstruction. Prophylactic ureteral stent placement before ESWL could be considered to help minimize the risk of ureteral obstruction and allow for passive ureteral dilation.[42,43] Transient hematuria is commonly seen. Pancreatitis is another reported complication and was documented in 2% to 3% of dogs.[44]

Although historically ESWL is thought to have minimal effect on the glomerular filtration rate (GFR) and the kidney itself, more recent reports in the human literature highlight short- and long-term effects that need to be considered before treatment. The repeated shockwaves necessary to cause stone fragmentation are also responsible for generating tissue damage, resulting in vascular hemorrhage. Dose-dependent renal fibrosis has been demonstrated in a canine experimental model.[45] Extracorporeal shockwave lithotripsy is contraindicated in patients that are coagulopathic. In addition, damage of surrounding tissues can occur, and in humans reported complications include: perforation of the colon, rupture of the hepatic artery, hepatic hematoma, pneumothorax, urinothorax, rupture of the spleen, acute necrotizing pancreatitis, dissecting abdominal wall abscess, rupture of the abdominal aorta, and iliac vein thrombosis.[46–58] These complications are very rare. Experimental models in pigs have shown that following certain protocols for energy settings and pulsing frequency, the injury can be reduced significantly.[59–66] Thus, ESWL is a viable option in our canine patients but should be performed by an experienced operator so that adverse side effects can be minimized.

In veterinary patients nephrolith size limitations are considered to avoid creating obstructive ureterolithiasis out of non-obstructive nephrolithiasis. The authors will always consider concurrent endoscopic ureteral stent placement before considering ESWL for this reason. The size limit for ESWL in the authors' practice is 1 to 1.5 cm in diameter. For stones larger than this, or composed of cystine, which are inherently ESWL resistant, an endoscopic nephrolithotomy is considered a better option.[40]

Endoscopic Nephrolithotomy

Endoscopic nephrolithotomy can be considered with large nephroliths over 1 to 1.5 cm in diameter, or those that are ESWL resistant (eg, cystine). When compared with ESWL, laparoscopic-assisted nephrotomy, and traditional nephrotomy, endoscopic nephrolithotomy is reported to be the most kidney-sparing procedure, likely due to the spreading rather than transection of the renal parenchyma at the access point (**Fig. 3**).[67–69]

The approach can be percutaneous nephrolithotomy (PCNL) or surgically assisted endoscopic nephrolithotomy (SENL). These 2 procedures are performed similarly, using endoscopic and fluoroscopic guidance. The percutaneous approach uses ultrasonic guidance to gain access into the renal pelvis from the greater curvature of the kidney.[70] An 18-gauge renal access needle is directed onto the pelvis, onto the nephroliths. Once access is obtained, a pyeloureterogram is performed so the guide wire can be advanced into the renal pelvis, down the ureter, into the urinary bladder, and out of the urethra. This acts as the safety wire so that through-and-through access is maintained throughout the procedure. A dilation sheath is then advanced over the guide wire so that a balloon catheter (typically 8 mm) may be used to dilate a tract from the skin, through the renal parenchyma and into the renal pelvis. The balloon is inflated to 8 mm (24 F) and a 24 F access sheath is then advanced over the inflated balloon using fluoroscopic guidance, and onto the stone. The balloon is then deflated and the sheath remains in place providing access for a nephroscope directly onto the stone (see **Fig. 3**). Using intracorporeal lithotripsy, the stone is fragmented and pieces are either suctioned or extracted until the renal pelvis is free of stone material. After removal of all stone fragments, a double pigtail ureteral stent is placed to ensure patency in the event of ureteral spasm or passage of any remaining small fragments of mineral debris. When performed percutaneously, a locking loop nephrostomy tube is then placed to allow a nephropexy to occur at the access site and to prevent development of a uroabdomen. This tube remains in place for 2 to 4 weeks at home.

When performing this technique with surgical assistance (SENL), the same approach is taken but a routine laparotomy is performed, and, on completion of ureteral stent placement, the stoma in the kidney is closed with a single mattress suture. No nephrostomy tube is left in place.

The main risks of this procedure include hemorrhage, ureteral perforation, and urine leakage from the renal access tract. Use of the balloon dilator and sheath combination, as described above, helps to tamponade any potential bleeding that could occur during access. These procedures are thought to be the most kidney-sparing option for large nephrolithotomy as the renal parenchyma is stretched rather than transected for stone removal. PCNL/SENL was recently reported in 11 dogs and 1 cat.[70] The authors in this study preferred to modify the technique from a PCNL to SENL to allow for closure of the renal tract, which was preferred by the owners at home and technically

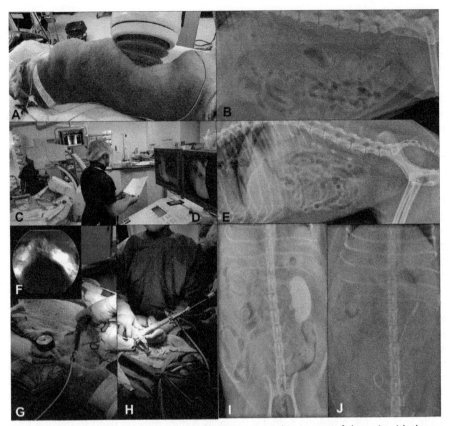

Fig. 3. (*A, C*) Positioning and monitoring for ESWL. Note the contact of the unit with the patient for appropriate conductivity. (*B, E*) Pre- and post-ESWL. Note stent placement to ensure patency while any fragments pass. (*D*) Note the continued monitoring via fluoroscopy during shockwave. (*F*) Endoscopic view of the renal pelvis during an SENL. (*G*) Balloon dilation to spread apart renal parenchyma and allow for placement of a nephroscope. (*H*) Positioning of the nephroscope and lithotripter. (*I, J*) Pre- and post-SENL.

provides a more caudolateral access point, expediting the procedure for stone removal and ensuring ureteral patency at completion. In this report, patient size was not seen to be a factor in success (range, 2.3–49 kg), but the appropriate equipment and proper training are necessary for a successful outcome.

Obstructive Ureterolithiasis

Ureteral obstructions are a serious condition in veterinary patients, and with the advent of high-quality imaging and awareness they are becoming more frequently diagnosed in our canine and feline patients. Because of kidney functional loss associated with the increased hydrostatic pressure of a ureteral obstruction, this condition does require timely intervention.[71–73] In an experimental model using dogs with no pre-existing azotemia, a complete ureteral obstruction resulted in an immediate increase in renal pelvic pressure, decreased renal blood flow by 60% within the first 24 hours, and acute decrease in the glomerular filtration rate.[71] After 7 days, GFR was permanently decreased by 35%, and after 2 weeks by 54%. In clinical patients, where kidney damage has likely already been done, no hypertrophic mechanisms occur to aid in kidney functional recovery, and a worse outcome would be expected.

The composition of most ureteroliths in dogs (50%–60%) and cats (>92%) are calcium based, making dissolution completely contraindicated in cats, and should not be considered in dogs with struvite stones that have not yet accomplished ureteral decompression.[4,74–76] With medical management being effective in few feline cases (8%–13%), and traditional surgical interventions being associated with a relatively high postoperative complication rate (30%–40% in cats and ~7%-15% in dogs) and perioperative mortality rate (18%–21% in cats and 6.25% in dogs), short-term medical therapy should be considered before any intervention (24–48 hours), if possible.[2,75–78]

The most common complications associated with surgery were due to ureterotomy site edema, re-obstruction from nephroliths that pass to the surgery site, stricture formation at the surgical site, missed ureteroliths not removed, and surgery-associated urine leakage.[2,75] Because of the high mortality rates and high complication rates, alternatives have been developed for animals over the past decade to avoid traditional open ureteral surgery.

Interventional alternatives have shown to result in immediate decompression, fewer peri-operative complications, lower peri-operative mortality rates, successful treatment for all causes of obstruction (stone, stricture, tumor), and a decreased recurrence rate of future obstructions, when compared with traditional options (40% with traditional surgery or medical management within 1 year).[4,74–76] The etiology of feline ureterolithiasis was recently shown to be associated with a ureteral stricture in approximately 33% of cases making surgical repair a far more complicated proposition.[4,76] Interventional therapies, like ureteral stents or the subcutaneous ureteral bypass (SUB) device are more amenable for all causes of ureteral obstructions.

Medical management for the treatment of ureterolith-induced obstructions typically uses a combination of intravenous fluid therapy and an alpha-adrenergic blockade with mannitol. In the authors' experience approximately 10% success is seen with medical management alone.

Ureteral Stenting

The use of double pigtail ureteral stents has been reported in dogs and cats with excellent outcomes as an alternative to traditional surgery.[4,74,78–82] Ureteral stent placement allows for immediate kidney decompression, a decreased risk for ureteral stricture and urine leakage after surgery, and a decrease rate of obstruction recurrence. In feline patients ureteral stenting improved the mortality associated with traditional surgery (7.2%), but was associated with a 38% rate of long-term dysuria, most of which resolved with steroid therapy.[4] Nineteen percent of ureteral stents in cats needed to be exchanged, most commonly due to re-obstruction from a ureteral stricture or ureteral stent migration. Since the advent of the SUB device, both the short- and long-term complications have improved for ureteral obstructions in cats, and ureteral stents have been more reserved for dogs, in the authors' practice.

In dogs, ureteral stents can most commonly be placed endoscopically and fluoroscopically guided.[74] Passive ureteral dilation has been reported to occur within 2 weeks of placement, and in this report the dilation was significant enough to allow for post-stenting ureteroscopy with a 3.1-mm ureteroscope within 2 weeks.[43] Complications are uncommon but include stent occlusion, compression, migration, and proliferative tissue at the ureterovesicular junction. Ureteral stents needed to be exchanged in 14% of dogs, and this was most commonly due to obstructive ureteritis (**Fig. 4**). In dogs, ureteral stents are typically outpatient procedures performed during retrograde cystourethroscopy. This is the authors' preferred treatment for obstructive pyonephrosis allowing for renal pelvic lavage and decompression of the obstructive lesion simultaneously, avoiding invasive surgery.[83]

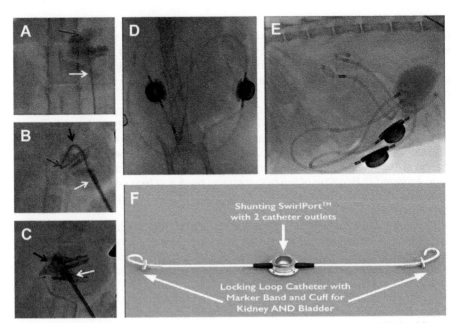

Fig. 4. Fluoroscopic images during placement of the SUB device. (*A*) A modified Seldinger technique is used to gain access to the renal pelvis. Note the guide wire (*red arrow*) being fed through an 18 g catheter (*white arrow*). (*B*) The 18 g catheter has been removed, and the nephrostomy tube (*black arrow*) is being fed over the guide wire (*red arrow*). Note the radiopaque marker (*white arrow*) that identifies the end of the fenestrations in the nephrostomy tube. (*C*) The guide wire has been removed and the pigtail (*black arrow*) has been locked in place. The radiopaque marker (*white arrow*) is positioned to ensure all fenestrations are within the renal pelvis. (*D*) Bilateral SUB with each nephrostomy catheter positioned so that is, going down the ureter rather than coiling the renal pelvis. This is preferred when there is a small degree of renal pelvic dilation. (*E*) Lateral view following bilateral SUB placement. Note the radiopaque markers on the cystostomy catheters are positioned inside the bladder. (*F*) A SUB device with 2 catheter outlets. This is preferred to a 3-way port in the case of any benign obstruction.

In most cases, retrograde stent placement via an endoscopic approach can be performed. In a study of 47 dogs with 57 ureters undergoing stent placement for various benign obstructions, long-term complications included urinary tract infection (26%), occlusion of the stent (9%), suspected ureteritis (5%), stent migration (5%), encrustation of the stent (2%), and hematuria (7%).[74] For the dogs experiencing infection postprocedure, all had infection present before stent placement and 72% were ultimately able to clear the infection.[74] If stones are suspected to be struvite, dissolution should be attempted following kidney decompression, and following dissolution the stent can be removed endoscopically.[74] If another stone type that is likely to be recurrent is suspected, the stent could be left in place long-term provided there are no complications. If stent exchange is indicated, the procedure can typically be performed on an outpatient basis.

Subcutaneous Ureteral Bypass Device

The SUB device is an artificial ureter that consists of a combination of a locking loop nephrostomy tube, a cystostomy tube, and a subcutaneously placed metallic shunting port that connects the 2 catheters (**Fig. 5**). This device allows urine to flow from the

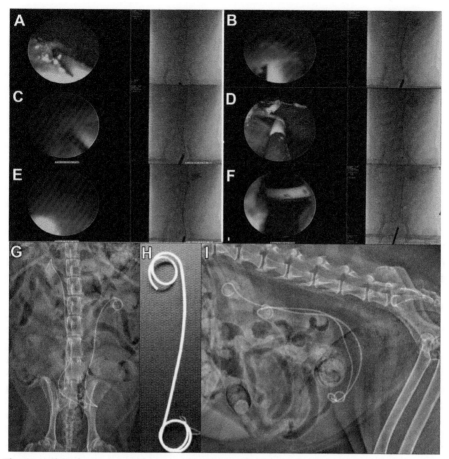

Fig. 5. *A–F)* Endoscopic and fluoroscopic retrograde placement of a ureteral stent in a dog. Note positioning of a guidewire into the ureteral orifice followed a ureteral marker catheter so that a ureteropyelogram can be performed in preparation for stent deployment. (*G, I*) Post-procedure radiographs confirming appropriate stent placement. (*H*) Example of a multi-fenestrated double -pigtail ureteral stent.

kidney to the urinary bladder without any manipulation of the ureter, avoiding the need to address the challenging underlying etiology (eg, stone(s), stricture, tumor, extraluminal compression) causing the ureteral obstruction.[83,84]

The use of the SUB device was recently reported for the treatment of benign ureteral obstructions 134 cats (174 ureters) with good to excellent outcomes.[76] In this population 33% of obstructions were due to strictures, 33% were bilaterally obstructed, and over 95% of cats were azotemic despite a unilateral ureteral obstruction. In this population the peri-operative mortality rate was 6.2%, the lowest for any procedure reported to date, and the median procedure time is 45 minutes. The median creatinine at presentation was 6.6 mg/dL and 2.4 mg/dL at the time of discharge. The overall mean survival time was 827 days, and the mean survival time for a non-renal cause of death was over 2251 days. There was no pre-operative predictor of long-term survival.

The most significant complication long-term was device mineralization (24%), with 13% developing a re-obstruction requiring a SUB device exchange. The other 11%

developed a patent ureter and were no longer obstructed despite a poorly flowing SUB device. Since the routine flushing protocol was performed using a tetra-EDTA solution, the mineralization rate declined to 4.5% (Berent, unpublished data collected between 2013 and 2017). Chronic urinary tract infections were seen in 8% of patients, and this was most common in cats that were infected before SUB device placement. Compared with feline ureteral stents, the SUB device was associated with dysuria in 8% of cats, most of which had a history of dysuria before their SUB placement.[76]

In the authors' practice, this device has essentially replaced the use of traditional surgery and double pigtail ureteral stents for the treatment of ureteral obstructions in feline patients. This is due to the combination of the ease of placement, the decreased rates of dysuria and re-obstruction, and the low peri-operative mortality.

The SUB device has also been used in a small group of dogs. A recent report showed that the SUB device in dogs was effective in relieving the ureteral obstruction in all cases, most of which were from a failed ureteral stent, but was associated with a 50% rate of device mineralization and ultimately SUB occlusion (Milligan M, Berent AC, Weisse C. Outcomes of SUB in dogs with benigng obstructions: 9 cases [2013-2017]. Unpublished data collected between 2013 and 2017). Because of this finding, and the low rate of ureteral stent occlusions, the authors prefer ureteral stents in dogs and the SUB device in cats.

SUMMARY

Interventional options for the treatment of upper urinary tract obstructions in veterinary medicine has dramatically expanded over the past decade, and is continuing to do so. This is following the trend that has been occurring in human medicine over the past 30 years, and will likely continue to grow in our profession as more clinicians are getting trained, more literature is being published to show evidence of superior methods evolving, and clients are demanding higher standards for their pets.

It is highly recommended that operators get proper training before considering all of the procedures described as the learning curve is steep and complications should be avoided whenever possible. Training laboratories are available to further develop these skills. In addition, treatment of stone disease should always consider the stone type and the ideal method for bypass, removal, or monitoring.

REFERENCES

1. Ling GV, Franti CE, Johnson BA, et al. Urolithasis in dogs II: breed prevalence, and interrelations of breed, sex, age, and mineral composition. Am J Vet Res 1998;9:630–43.
2. Snyder DM, Steffey MA, Mehler SJ, et al. Diagnosis and surgical management of ureteral calculi in dogs: 16 cases (1990-2003). N Z Vet J 2005;53(1):19–25.
3. Ross SJ, Osborne CA, Lulich JP, et al. Canine and feline nephrolithiasis: epidemiology, detection and management. Vet Clin North Am Small Amin Pract 1999;29: 231–50.
4. Berent A, Weisse C, Bagley D. Ureteral stenting for benign feline ureteral obstructions: technical and clinical outcomes in 79 ureters (2006-2010). J Am Vet Med Assoc 2014;244:559–76.
5. Bartges JW, Oscorne CA, Pozin DJ. Recurrent sterile struvite urolithasis in three related cocker spaniels. J Am Anim Hosp Assoc 1992;28:459–69.
6. Osborne CA, Lulich JP, Kruger JM, et al. Medical dissolution of feline struvite urocystoliths. J Am Vet Med Assoc 1990;196:1053–63.

7. Cannon AB, Westropp JL, Ruby AL, et al. Evaluation of trends in uroliths composition in cats: 5230 cases (1985-2004). J Am Vet Med Assoc 2007;231(4):570–6.

8. Abdullahi SU, Osborne CA, Leininger JR, et al. Evaluation of a calculolytic diet in female dogs with induced struvite urolithasis. Am J Vet Res 1984;45:1508–19.

9. McLean RJ, Nickel JC, Beveridge TJ, et al. Observations of the ultrastructure of infected kidney stones. J Med Microbiol 1989;29(2):1–7.

10. Bannasch D, Safra N, Young A, et al. Mutations in the SLC2A9 gene cause hyperuricosuria and hyperuricemia in the dog. PLoS Genet 2008;4(11):e1000246. Barsh GS, ed.

11. Karmi N, Safra N, Young A, et al. Validation of a urine test and characterization of the putative genetic mutation for hyperuricosuria in Bulldogs and Black Russian Terriers. Am J Vet Res 2010;71(8):909–14.

12. Bartges JW, Osborne CA, Felice LJ, et al. Diet effect on activity product ratios of uric acid sodium urate, and ammonium urate in urine formed by healthy beagles. Am J Vet Res 1995;6:329–33.

13. Dear JD, Shiraki R, Ruby A, et al. Feline urate urolithasis: a retrospective study of 159 cases. J Feline Med Surg 2011;13(10):725–32.

14. Bartges JW, Osborne CA, Koehler LA, et al. An algorithmic approach to canine urate urolthiasis. etiopathogenesis, diagnosis, treatment, and prevention. Vet Clin North Am Small Anim Pract 1999;29:193–211.

15. Bartges JW, Osborne CA, Felice LJ, et al. Bioavailability and pharmacokinetics of intravenously and orally administered allopurinol to healthy dogs. Am J Vet Res 1997;58:504–10.

16. Westropp JL, Larsen JA, Johnson EG, et al. Evaluation of dogs with genetic hyperuricosuria and urate urolithiasis consuming a purine restricted diet: a pilot study. BMC Vet Res 2017;13(1):45.

17. Ling GV, Ruby AL, Harrold DR, et al. Xanthine-containing urinary calculi in dogs given allopurinol. J Am Vet Med Assoc 1991;198:195–1940.

18. Nakagawa Y, Asplin JR, Goldfarb DS, et al. Clinical use of cystine supersaturation measurements. J Urol 2000;164:1482–5.

19. Osborne CA, Sanderson SL, Lulich JP, et al. Canine cystine uroithasis: cause, detecton, treatment, and prevention. Vet Clin North Am Small Anim Pract 1999;29: 193–211.

20. Brons AK, Henthorn PS, Raj K, et al. SLC3A1 and SLC7A9 mutations in autosomal recessive or dominant canine cystinuria: a new classification system. J Vet Intern Med 2013;27(6):1400–8.

21. Henthorn PS, Liu J, Gidalevich T, et al. Canine cystinuria: polymorphism in the canine SLC3A1 gene and identification of a nonsense mutation in cystinuric Newfoundland dogs. Hum Genet 2000;107:295–303.

22. Asplin DM, Asplin JR. The interaction of thiol drugs and urine pH in the treatment of cystinuria. J Urol 2013;189:2147–51.

23. Robertson WB, Jones JS, Heaton MA, et al. Predicting the crystallization potential of urine from cats and dogs with respect to calcium oxalate and magnesium ammonium phosphate (struvite). J Nutr 2002;132:1637S–41S.

24. Ling GV, Thurmond MC, Choi YK, et al. Change in proportion of canine urinary calculi composed of calcium oxalate or struvite in specimens analyzed from 1981-2001. J Vet Intern Med 2003;17:817–23.

25. Albasan H, Osborne CA, Lulich JP, et al. Rate and frequency of recurrence of ammonium urate, calcium oxalate, and struvite uroliths in cats. J Am Vet Med Assoc 2009;235:1450–5.

26. Okafor CC, Lefebvre, Pearl DL. Risk factors associated with calcium oxalate ur-olithasis in dogs evaluated at general care veterinary hospital in the United States. Prev Vet Med 2014;115:217–28.

27. Lekcharoensuk C, Osborne CA, Lulich JP, et al. Associations between dry dietary factors and canine calcium oxalate uroliths. Am J Vet Res 2002;63:330–7.

28. Kaul P, Sidhu H, Sharma SK, et al. Calculogenic potential of galactose and fruc-tose in relation to urinary excretion of lithogenic substances in vitamin B6 defi-cient and control rats. J Am Coll Nutr 1996;15(3):295–302.

29. Gnanandarajah JS, Abrahante JE, Lulich JP, et al. Presence of Oxalobacter for-migenes in the intestinal tract is associated with the absence of calcium oxalate urolith formation in dogs. Urol Res 2012;40(5):467–73.

30. Stevenson AE, Wrigglesworth DJ, Smith BH, et al. Effects of dietary potassium cit-rate supplementation on urine pH and urinary relative supersaturation of calcium oxalate and struvite in healthy dogs. Am J Vet Res 2000;61:430–5.

31. Hezel A, Bartges JW, Kirk CA, et al. Influence of hydrochlorothiazide on urinay calcium oxalate relative supersaturation in healthy young adult female domestic shorthaired cats. Vet Ther 2007;8:247–54.

32. Lulich JP, Osborne CA, Lekcharoensuk C, et al. Effects of hydrochlorothiazide and diet in dogs with calcium oxalate urolithasis. J Am Vet Med Assoc 2001; 218:1583–6.

33. Bolliger C, Walshaw R, Kruger JM, et al. Evaluation of the effect of nephrotomy on renal function in clinically normal cats. Am J Vet Res 2005;66(8):1400–7.

34. King M, Waldron D, Barber D, et al. Effect of nephrotomy on renal function and morphology in normal cats. Vet Surg 2006;35(8):749–58.

35. Gookin JL, Stone EA, Spaulding KA, et al. Unilateral nephrectomy in dogs with renal disease: 30 cases (1985-1994). J Am Vet Med Assoc 1996;208(12):2020–6.

36. Lulich JP, Berent AC, Adams LG, et al. ACVIM small animal consensus recom-mendations on the treatment and prevention of uroliths in dogs and cats. J Vet Intern Med 2016;30(5):1564–74.

37. Adams LG, Goldman CK. Extracorporeal shock wave lithotripsy. In: Polzin DJ, Bartges JB, editors. Nephrology and urology of small animals. Ames (IA): Black-well Publishing; 2011. p. 340–8.

38. Adams LG, Williams JC Jr, McAteer JA, et al. In vitro evaluation of canine and fe-line urolith fragility by shock wave lithotripsy. Am J Vet Res 2005;66:1651–4.

39. Adams LG. Nephroliths and ureteroliths: a new stone age. N Z Vet J 2013;61(4): 212–6.

40. Williams JC Jr, Saw KC, Paterson RF, et al. Variability of renal stone fragility in shock wave lithotripsy. Urology 2003;61:1092–7.

41. Block G, Adams LG, Widmer WR, et al. Use of extracorporeal shock wave litho-tripsy for treatment of nephrolithiasis and ureterolithiasis in five dogs. J Am Vet Med Assoc 1996;208:531–6.

42. Hubert KC, Palmar JS. Passive dilation by ureteral stenting before ureteroscopy: eliminating the need for active dilation. J Urol 2005;174(3):1079–80.

43. Vachon C, Defarges A, Berent A, et al. Passive ureteral dilation and ureterosocpy following ureteral stent placement in normal dogs. Am J Vet Res 2017;78(3): 381–92.

44. Daugherty MA, Adams LG, Baird DK, et al. Acute pancreatitis in two dogs asso-ciated with shock wave lithotripsy [abstract]. J Vet Intern Med 2004;18:441.

45. Newman R, Hackett R, Senior D, et al. Pathological effects of ESWL on canine renal tissue. Urology 1987;29:194–200.

46. Castillon I, Frieyro O, Gonzalez-Enguita C, et al. Colonic perforation after extra-corporeal shock wave lithotripsy. BJU Int 1999;83:720–1.
47. Beatrice J, Strebel RT, Pfammatter T, et al. Life-threatening complication after right renal extracorporeal shock wave lithotripsy: large hepatic haematoma requiring embolisation of the right hepatic artery. Eur Urol 2007;52:909–11.
48. Fugita OE, Trigo-Rocha F, Mitre AI, et al. Splenic rupture and abscess after extra-corporeal shock wave lithotripsy. Urology 1998;52:322–3.
49. Karakayali F, Sevmi S, Ayvaz I, et al. Acute necrotizing pancreatitis as a rare complication of extracorporeal shock wave lithotripsy. Int J Urol 2006;13:613–5.
50. Hassan I, Zietlow SP. Acute pancreatitis after extracorporeal shock wave litho-tripsy for a renal calculus. Urology 2002;60:1111.
51. Oguzulgen IK, Oguzulgen AI, Sinik Z, et al. An unusual cause of urinothorax. Respiration 2002;69:273–4.
52. Unal B, Kara S, Bilgili Y, et al. Giant abdominal wall abscess dissecting into thorax as a complication of ESWL. Urology 2005;65:389e16-18.
53. Neri E, Capannini G, Diciolla F, et al. Localized dissection and delayed rupture of the abdominal aorta after extracorporeal shock wave lithotripsy. J Vasc Surg 2000;31:1052–5.
54. Tiede JM, Lumpkin EN, Wass CT, et al. Hemoptysis following extracorporeal shock wave lithotripsy: a case of lithotripsy-induced pulmonary contusion in a pe-diatric patient. J Clin Anesth 2003;15:530–3.
55. Meyer JJ, Cass AS. Subcapsular hematoma of the liver after renal extracorporeal shock wave lithotripsy. J Urol 1995;154:516–7.
56. Malhotra V, Rosen RJ, Slepian RL. Life-threatening hypoxemia after lithotripsy in an adult due to shock-wave-induced pulmonary contusion. Anesthesiology 1991; 75:529–31.
57. Gayer G, Hertz M, Stav K, et al. Minimally invasive management of urolithiasis. Semin Ultrasound CT MR 2007;27:139–51.
58. Skolarikos A, Alivizatos G, de la Rosette J. Extracorporeal shock wave lithotripsy 25years later: complications and their prevention. Eur Urol 2006;50:981–90.
59. Evan AP, McAteer JA, Connors BA, et al. Renal injury in SWL is significantly reduced by slowing the rate of shock wave delivery. BJU Int 2007;100(3):624–7.
60. Willis LR, Evan AP, Connors BA, et al. Shockwave lithotripsy: dose-related effects on renal structure, hemodynamics, and tubular function. J Endourol 2005;19: 90–101.
61. Connors BA, Evan AP, Blomgren PM, et al. Reducing shock number dramatically decreases lesion size in a juvenile kidney model. J Endourol 2006;20:607–11.
62. Connors BA, Evan AP, Willis LR, et al. The effect of discharge voltage on renal injury and impairment caused by lithotripsy in the pig. J Am Soc Nephrol 2000; 11:310–8.
63. Delius M, Enders G, Xuan ZR, et al. Biological effects of shock waves: kidney damage by shock waves in dogs–dose dependence. Ultrasound Med Biol 1988;14:117–22.
64. Delius M, Enders G, Xuan ZR, et al. Biological effects of shock waves: kidney haemorrhage by shock waves in dogs–administration rate dependence. Ultra-sound Med Biol 1988;14:689–94.
65. Delius M, Mueller W, Goetz A, et al. Biological effects of shock waves: kidney hemorrhage in dogs at a fast shock wave administration rate of fifteen Hertz. J Lithotr Stone Dis 1990;2:103–10.

66. Evan AP, McAteer JA, Connors BA, et al. Independent assessment of a wide-focus, low-pressure electromagnetic lithotripter: absence of renal bioeffects in the pig. BJU Int 2008;101(3):382–8.

67. Meretyk S, Gofrit ON, Gafni O, et al. Complete staghorn calculi: random prospective comparison between extracorporeal shock wave lithotripsy monotherapy and combined with percutaneous nephrostolithotomy. J Urol 1997;157:780–6.

68. Al-Hunayan A, Khalil M, Hassabo M, et al. Management of solitary renal pelvic stone: laparoscopic retroperitoneal pyelolithotomy versus percutaneous nephrolithotomy. J Endourol 2011;25(6):975–8.

69. Chen KK, Chen MT, Yeh SH, et al. Radionuclide renal function study in various surgical treatments of upper urinary stones. Zhonghua Yi Xue Za Zhi (Taipei) 1992;49(5):319–27.

70. Petrovsky B, Berent AC, Weisse CW, et al. Endoscopic nephrolithotomy for the removal of complicated nephrolithiasis in11 dogs and 1 cat (2005-2017), in press.

71. Fink RW, Caradis DT, Chmiel R, et al. Renal impairment and its reversibility following variable periods of complete ureteric obstruction. Aust N Z J Surg 1980;50:77–83.

72. Kerr WS. Effect of complete ureteral obstruction for one week on kidney function. J Appl Physiol 1954;6:762.

73. Vaughan DE, Sweet RE, Gillenwater JY. Unilateral ureteral occlusion: pattern of nephron repair and compensatory response. J Urol 1973;109:979.

74. Pavia PR, Berent AC, Weisse CW, et al. Outcome of ureteral stent placement for treatment of benign ureteral obstruction in dogs: 44 cases (2010–2013). JAVMA 2018;252(6):721–31.

75. Kyles A, Hardie E, Wooden E, et al. Management and outcome of cats with ureteral calculi: 153 cases (1984–2002). J Am Vet Med Assoc 2005;226(6):937–44.

76. Berent A, Weisse C, Bagley D, et al. The use of a subcutaneous ureteral bypass device for the treatment of feline ureteral obstructions. Seville (Spain): ECVIM; 2011.

77. Roberts S, Aronson L, Brown D. Postoperative mortality in cats after ureterolithotomy. Vet Surg 2011;40:438–43.

78. Wormser C, Clarke DL, Aronson LR. Outcomes of ureteral surgery and ureteral stenting in cats: 117 cases (2006-2014). J Am Vet Med Assoc 2016;248(5):518–25.

79. Berent A, Weisse C, Beal M, et al. Use of indwelling, double-pigtail stents for treatment of malignant ureteral obstruction in dogs: 12 cases (2006-2009). J Am Vet Med Assoc 2011;238(8):1017–25.

80. Horowitz C, Berent A, Weisse C, et al. Predictors of outcome for cats with ureteral obstructions after interventional management using ureteral stents or a subcutaneous ureteral bypass device. J Feline Med Surg 2013;15(12):1052–62.

81. Kuntz J, Berent A, Weisse C, et al. Double pigtail ureteral stenting and renal pelvic lavage for renal-sparing treatment of pyonephrosis in dogs: 13 cases (2008-2012). J Am Vet Med Assoc 2015;246(2):216–25.

82. Lam N, Berent A, Weisse C, et al. Ureteral stenting for congenital ureteral strictures in a dog. J Am Vet Med Assoc 2012;240(8):983–90.

83. Steinhaus J, Berent AC, Weisse C, et al. Clinical presentation and outcome of cats with circumcaval ureters associated with a ureteral obstruction. J Vet Intern Med 2014;29(1):63–70.

84. Zaid M, Berent A, Weisse C, et al. Feline ureteral strictures: 10 cases (2007-2009). J Vet Intern Med 2011;25(2):222–9.

Nutritional Management of Urolithiasis

Yann Queau, DVM

KEYWORDS

- Urolithiasis • Stone • Struvite • Calcium oxalate • Urate • Xanthine • Cystine
- Silica

KEY POINTS

- Dietary management of urolithiasis is designed to dissolve calculi (struvite, urate, cystine) and/or reduce the risk of recurrence.
- For mixed or compound stones, the dietary therapy should be based on the salt present in the nidus.
- For all types of stones, emphasis should be put on promoting urine dilution, which is best achieved by feeding high-moisture diets when possible.
- Controlling the amounts of crystal precursors in the diet as well as urine pH is important for all stones, although not clearly established for calcium oxalate.

INTRODUCTION

Uroliths are concretions that can form anywhere in the urinary tract, causing lower urinary tract signs if located in the bladder and urethra, or potentially acute or chronic kidney injury when located in the renal pelvises or ureters. Nutritional management is designed to dissolve urinary stones (struvite, urate, cystine) and/or reduce the risk of recurrence. The nature of the stone (suspected, or confirmed by quantitative analysis), its localization, the presence of potential comorbidities or underlying metabolic disorders, and the patient's history and environment are essential points to consider in order to guide and optimize dietary management.

Most stones occur as pure uroliths, and up to 11% may occur as compound or mixed uroliths.[1–3] In that case, dietary prevention should target the inner part of the calculus (nidus), which forms first and facilitates the precipitation of the second mineral.

Assessing the Risk of Crystallization in Urine

Uroliths are polycrystalline structures that form under certain conditions affecting the concentrations of crystalloids, inhibitors or promoters of crystallization, and pH.

Disclosure: The author is an employee of Royal Canin, a division of Mars, Inc.
Research & Development Center, Royal Canin, 650 avenue de la Petite Camargue, Aimargues 30470, France
E-mail address: yann.queau@royalcanin.com

Relative supersaturation (RSS) is a risk index of crystallization in humans and companion animals.[4,5] To calculate RSS, urine pH and the concentrations of 10 solutes from a representative urine sample are entered in a computer algorithm. RSS defines 3 levels of urine saturation: undersaturation (crystal dissolution, RSS<1 for struvite and calcium oxalate [CaOx]), metastable supersaturation (no spontaneous crystal formation or dissolution, RSS 1–2.5 for struvite and 1–12 for CaOx), and labile supersaturation (spontaneous crystal formation and growth).[5] Another CaOx risk index has been developed in humans (Bonn risk index[5]) and dogs and cats (CaOx titration test[6]) to take into account organic promoters and inhibitors of crystallization, but it is less specific because it only measures urinary calcium, and it currently lacks peer-reviewed publications in dogs and cats.

To date, RSS or other risk indices are not available in the clinical setting. Urine specific gravity (USG), urine pH, and microscopic evaluation can be readily performed as indirect and imperfect ways of assessing the risk of crystallization. Maintaining USG less than 1.030 in cats and less than 1.020 in dogs is therefore often recommended in patients at risk.[7]

General Considerations for All Uroliths: Stimulating Diuresis

Urine dilution is the paramount strategy for the prevention and/or the dissolution of all uroliths. Increased diuresis decreases the concentration of crystal precursors and stimulates more frequent urination, decreasing the time for crystal aggregation. Feeding wet diets exclusively (dietary moisture >70%) is an effective way to enhance water intake and diuresis in dogs and cats.[8–10] This effect is only seen in diets with greater than 70% moisture. Therefore, adding some wet diet only as a portion of a dry diet does not promote urine dilution; however, warm water can be poured onto kibbles: adding 1.5 cups of water to 1 cup of kibbles yields approximately 80% moisture. Acceptance of such diets might be a challenge but pets can be habituated progressively (**Fig. 1**).

When exclusively feeding a wet diet is not possible, sodium chloride supplementation is an alternative, although this does not provide as much dilution as a high-moisture diet.[7] In a large number of studies, cats and dogs had greater water intake and urine volume, and in most cases lower USG when fed dry commercial diets with sodium content greater than 2.5 g/1000 kcal.[10–18] The use of high dietary sodium

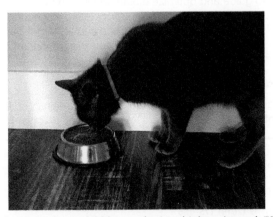

Fig. 1. Water can be poured onto kibbles to obtain a high-moisture (>70%) diet and promote urine dilution. (*Courtesy of* J.D. Dear, DVM, MAS; University of California, Davis.)

is subject to controversy. Based on human studies, concerns have been raised regarding kidney function, cardiac function, and blood pressure. One study found a reversible increase in creatinine level in 4 cats with marginally impaired kidney function when fed a diet with sodium at 2.9 g/1000 kcal.[16] In contrast, 5 short-term[19–22] (1–12 weeks) and 2 long-term[17,18,23,24] (6–24 months) studies found no effect of a higher sodium intake on kidney (including glomerular filtration rate) and cardiac functions in dogs or cats. Systemic hypertension was not found in any study.

Specific Considerations According to Stone Type

Struvite

Struvite crystals are composed of magnesium, ammonium, and phosphate. They can form in sterile urine (most feline cases) or secondary to a urinary tract infection (UTI) with urease-producing bacteria (most, if not all, canine cases). With urease-producing bacteria, ammonia is released from urea and urine is alkalinized, overcoming the effect of an acidifying diet. Therefore, the goals of dietary management for struvite depend on the species: prevention and dissolution in cats, and dissolution in dogs.

Roles of dietary precursors, urine dilution, and pH High dietary levels of phosphorus and magnesium increase their urinary excretion and the risk of struvite in cats[25–27]; however, urine dilution and pH are more important determinants of struvite formation. Urine dilution is effective to obtain a low struvite RSS (**Fig. 2**), as is an acidic urine pH. Results from trials in which healthy cats were fed dry diets of various nutrient profiles for 2 weeks show that urine pH<6.2 promotes an RSS less than 1 (see **Fig. 2**). In alkaline urine, phosphate is in its trivalent state (PO_4^{3-}), making it readily available to form struvite crystals ($NH_4MgPO_4 \cdot 6H_2O$), but, when urine is acidified, protonation of phosphate (HPO_4^{2-}, $H_2PO_4^-$, or H_3PO_4) decreases its availability. The acidification potential of a diet depends on its ingredients and the balance between acidifiers (eg, methionine, calcium or sodium sulfate, ammonium chloride) or alkalizers (eg, calcium

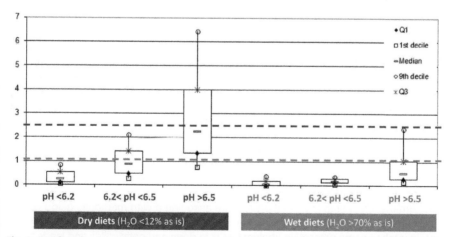

Fig. 2. Median (and deciles) struvite RSS according to urinary pH categories obtained for 481 dry diets and 27 wet diets in 142 adult cats. The green dashed line represents the solubility product for RSS struvite (limit between the undersaturated and the supersaturated zones) and the red dashed line represents the formation product (limit between the metastable and the labile supersaturation zones). (*Data from* Royal Canin cattery, Aimargues, France.)

carbonate, potassium citrate). Consumption of small meals throughout the day rather than 1 or 2 large meals blunts the postprandial alkaline tide and is associated with more acidic urine production and less struvite crystalluria.[28] The target urine pH to manage struvite uroliths is generally 6.0 to 6.3 (dry diets). Excessive chronic acidification increases urinary potassium excretion and the risk of body potassium depletion if dietary potassium is too low.[29,30] It could also promote bone demineralization, although this is not supported by studies in cats.[31–33]

Practical dietary management When struvite uroliths are suspected, medical dissolution is indicated before surgical removal, except in uncontrollable UTI.[7] Dry and canned veterinary commercial diets with controlled amounts of precursors, and acidifying and/or diuretic properties, successfully dissolve naturally occurring struvite uroliths in cats.[34–38] Average dissolution times were typically around 30 days, but complete dissolution time ranged from 6 to 141 days, which may be affected by the diet used and/or the size of the cystolith on starting the trial. Dissolution failures were caused by stones other than struvite. In dogs, dissolution can take up to 3 months, and protocols must be accompanied by appropriate antibiotic therapy.[39–41]

Calcium oxalate

CaOx uroliths are not amenable to medical dissolution. The goal of dietary management is to reduce the risk of recurrence.

Roles of urine dilution, dietary precursors, and pH Increasing water intake through dietary moisture[8,10,42] or dietary sodium[10–15,42,43] decreases CaOx RSS in healthy and stone-forming animals in most studies. A concern raised with high-sodium diets is an increased urinary calcium excretion.[11,13] However, because of concurrent urine dilution, urine calcium concentration is either unchanged[10,11,13,44] or decreased.[14] The urine concentrations of solutes such as oxalate can decrease, thus decreasing CaOx RSS.[10,11,14]

The role of dietary precursors in the pathophysiology of CaOx is poorly understood. Higher dietary moisture, protein, sodium, and potassium levels were retrospectively associated with a lower risk of CaOx in cats.[27] In dogs fed dry and canned diets, the risk of CaOx was higher for diets with the lowest levels of protein, sodium, potassium, calcium, phosphorus, and magnesium.[43,45,46] High-calcium levels increase its absorption (also affected by dietary phosphorus, magnesium, oxalate, and vitamin D) and urinary excretion, which lead to higher RSS,[47] so moderate levels are recommended. The effect of dietary oxalate (contained in ingredients such as beets, beans, potatoes, and leafy vegetables) on its urinary excretion is variable.[47–49] Oxalate absorption is also affected by dietary calcium[50] and intestinal oxalate-degrading bacteria. In addition, urinary oxalate excretion is influenced by endogenous production via the metabolism of some sugars (glucose, fructose), amino acids (eg, hydroxyproline, glycine, serine), or vitamin C.[48,49,51] Deficiency in vitamin B_6 (pyridoxine) increases endogenous production and excretion of oxalate[52] but is rare, and supplementation does not decrease oxaluria.[53]

In humans, diets high in animal protein are associated with metabolic acidosis and hypercalciuria[54] and are considered a risk factor for CaOx. In contrast, high dietary protein intake seems protective against CaOx in dogs and cats[27,45,46] and leads to increase urine volumes.[55–57] In cats, one study found slightly higher CaOx RSS with increasing dietary protein (35%–57% dry matter) in dry diets[58] but not in wet diets.[57] In addition, increasing protein was not associated with a consistent increase in calcium excretion or a decrease in urinary pH in either study.[57,58]

The effect of urine pH on the risk of CaOx remains controversial. The increasing prevalence of CaOx stones has been hypothesized to be associated with the general acidification of pet foods in the 1980s and 1990s. Retrospective epidemiologic studies have found urine-acidifying potential of diet (pH<6.25) to be associated with an increased risk of CaOx in cats[27] but not in dogs.[45,46,59] Chronic metabolic acidosis is thought to promote release of calcium and phosphate from bone and calciuria,[29,60] although this has been an inconsistent finding,[30,32] and to decrease urinary citrate, an inhibitor of CaOx crystallization. Controlled studies on the effect of acid urine pH on CaOx RSS have yielded conflicting results, showing either higher RSS despite similar ionized calcium and calciuria[33] or no difference in RSS.[61] In healthy cats fed dry and wet diets of various nutritional composition for periods of 2 weeks, CaOx RSS is not affected by urine pH (**Fig. 3**). Potassium citrate (75 mg/kg by mouth every 12–24 hours) is often recommended to decrease the risk of CaOx by alkalinizing urine and increasing citraturia,[7] but this strategy is not supported by 1 study in healthy dogs.[62] The optimal dose and clinical benefit therefore remain to be defined.

Practical management Dietary management of CaOx is designed to limit recurrence once stones have been removed surgically, or prevent further growth when removal is not possible or indicated (eg, nonproblematic nephroliths). It is also important to investigate and treat underlying metabolic disorders that could have promoted crystallization in the first place. Increased urinary calcium is a common feature of stone-forming dogs and cats,[63,64] and hypercalcemia should therefore be explored.

Several commercial diets are formulated with various strategies for the management of CaOx (eg, high dietary sodium, addition of potassium citrate) and have usually been tested in healthy animals to decrease CaOx RSS. Feline diets are typically acidifying to avoid the concurrent risk of struvite. However, there are currently insufficient prospective studies evaluating the efficacy of those diets to limit recurrence in stone-forming animals. One 2-year study in cats showed no significant difference between 2 diets that differed in calcium and magnesium contents and in urinary pH potential.[65] In a retrospective study, stone-forming dogs fed a high-sodium, acidifying diet (dry or canned) marketed for CaOx management had lower recurrence over time than a group of dogs fed any other diet.[66] Both studies, as well as previous data, suggest that,

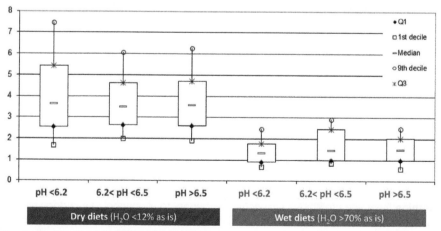

Fig. 3. Median (and deciles) CaOx RSS according to urinary pH categories obtained for 481 dry diets and 27 wet diets in 142 adult cats. (*Data from* Royal Canin cattery, Aimargues, France.)

despite diet modification, recurrence rate in animals with CaOx is high: 33% at 2 years in cats[65] and up to 57% at 3 years in dogs.[67] After stone removal, feeding a canned urinary diet exclusively remains the best recommendation. When this is not possible (owner or pet preference), a dry urinary diet (with added water as described earlier if accepted by the pet) is recommended. For CaOx nephroliths, a diet formulated for kidney disease is indicated in cases of concurrent kidney disease.

Calcium phosphate

When calcium phosphate uroliths occur as a minor component of CaOx or struvite stones, the management should be directed toward the original urolith (nidus). Pure calcium phosphate stones are associated with metabolic disorders leading to hypercalciuria (eg, hypercalcemia, hyperparathyroidism) and/or alkaline urine pH (eg, renal tubular acidosis).[68] These uroliths are not amenable to medical dissolution. Treating the underlying cause should be the first step to reduce the risk of recurrence. Diet should promote urine dilution (see earlier); contain controlled amounts of calcium, phosphorus, and vitamin D; and induce a moderately acid urine pH. Practically, most commercial diets marketed for the management of CaOx stones are formulated to achieve those goals.

Purine uroliths

Urate Dietary management of urate uroliths focuses primarily on preventing recurrent episodes in susceptible dogs (SLC2A9 mutation, portosystemic shunt) and cats. Medical dissolution has been reported in Dalmatians,[69] but not in dogs with uncorrected shunts or in cats.[7]

   Roles of dietary precursors, urine dilution, and pH As for other uroliths, urine dilution by promoting water intake should be the first step. Urinary urate results from the catabolism of endogenous or dietary purines (**Fig. 4**). Decreasing the purine content of the diet is effective to decrease urinary purine metabolites excretion.[70] Very-low-protein diets have been recommended to reduce 24-hour urinary excretion of uric acid.[71,72] However, the purine content of proteins varies (eg, it is high in organ meats and fish). By using selected protein sources (plant, egg white), severe restriction is not mandatory to achieve a low urinary urate level.[70,73] Urate crystals are slightly less soluble in acid urine. Therefore, the diet should not promote acid urine.

   Practical management In dogs, a few commercial diets with different nutritional profiles (protein levels and sources) and low in purines have been evaluated in dogs with the SLC2A9 mutation, for their effect on urinary urate excretion and/or stone recurrence.[73–75] Water can be added to the dry diets to encourage urine dilution (see earlier).[73] Allopurinol (5-7 mg/kg per mouth every 12 to 24 hours), which inhibits the conversion of hypoxanthine to uric acid, can be administered to dogs in conjunction with purine-restricted diets to decrease urate excretion.[7] In dogs with uncorrected portosystemic shunts and hepatic encephalopathy, a diet designed for liver disease may be advised. Homemade diets with low-purine protein sources and sufficient moisture content are an option but should be formulated by a veterinary nutritionist to be balanced. No dietary study has been conducted in cats, and diets designed for kidney or liver disease, which are typically protein restricted, are currently recommended.

Xanthine Xanthine uroliths usually occur secondary to allopurinol use in dogs fed diets high in purines (see **Fig. 4**), but can also occur spontaneously. No medical dissolution has been reported. Preventing recurrence of xanthine stones relies on adjustment of allopurinol dose and a similar but strict dietary strategy as for urate uroliths.

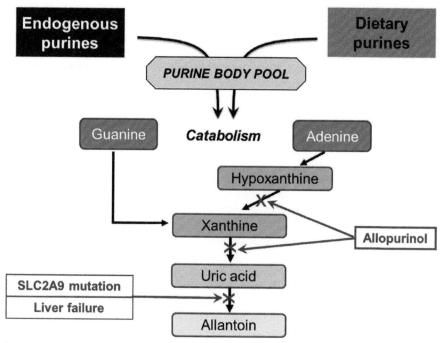

Fig. 4. Purine metabolism. In normal dogs and cats, allantoin, soluble in urine, is the main end product.

Cystine

For cystine stones, dietary treatment should be designed to dissolve them and prevent recurrence.[7] Again, promoting urine dilution is of paramount importance. Urine cystine excretion can be modulated by dietary protein intake, and more specifically methionine and cysteine.[76,77] Feeding a diet containing amounts of these essential amino acids close to their minimum requirements is therefore recommended. Most plant protein sources have smaller amounts of sulfur amino acids than animal proteins. The solubility of cystine is highly dependent on pH, with higher solubility for pH>7.2.[78] A low-protein alkalinizing diet and/or medical treatment with 2-mercaptopropionylglycine (2-MPG) (15–20 mg/kg by mouth every 12 hours) has been successfully used in dogs.[77,79] In cystinuric dogs, carnitinuria and taurine deficiency have been reported,[80] and taurine and carnitine are advised to prevent dilated cardiomyopathy, especially if fed diets restricted in their precursor methionine.

Silica

Silica uroliths are uncommon in dogs and cats, and medical dissolution has never been reported. For prevention, emphasis should be put on urine dilution. Preventing pica, avoiding diets rich in high-silica plant ingredients (eg, brown rice or soybean hulls), and offering bottled water in areas with soils high in silica are recommended. Canned diets, aside from promoting diuresis, are typically lower in vegetable ingredients. The effect of urine pH on silica solubility is unknown.

SUMMARY

Diet is a fundamental aspect of the management of urolithiasis in dogs and cats after individual risk factors have been identified. Success of the dietary management requires proper identification of the urolith, the management of metabolic disturbances, and compliance of the owner with the diet. Promoting water intake and urine dilution is a common feature regardless of cause. The management of some uroliths (struvite, urate, cystine) relies strongly on a specific dietary profile that controls dietary precursors and/or urinary pH. Most research in dogs and cats has been concerned with the mineral aspect of crystal formation, and more studies are required to investigate the importance of organic promoters and inhibitors. Because recurrence rate can be high for some types of uroliths and some patients, regular monitoring (urinalysis and imaging) is key to adjusting dietary therapy as needed.

REFERENCES

1. Osborne CA, Lulich JP, Kruger JM, et al. Analysis of 451,891 canine uroliths, feline uroliths, and feline urethral plugs from 1981 to 2007: perspectives from the Minnesota Urolith Center. Vet Clin North Am Small Anim Pract 2009;39(1):183–97.

2. Houston DM, Vanstone NP, Moore AE, et al. Evaluation of 21 426 feline bladder urolith submissions to the Canadian Veterinary Urolith Centre (1998-2014). Can Vet J 2016;57(2):196–201.

3. Houston DM, Weese HE, Vanstone NP, et al. Analysis of canine urolith submissions to the Canadian Veterinary Urolith Centre, 1998-2014. Can Vet J 2017; 58(1):45–50.

4. Robertson WG, Jones JS, Heaton MA, et al. Predicting the crystallization potential of urine from cats and dogs with respect to calcium oxalate and magnesium ammonium phosphate (struvite). J Nutr 2002;132(6 Suppl 2):1637S–41S.

5. Bartges J. Urinary saturation testing. In: Bartges J, Polzin DJ, editors. Nephrology and urology of small animals. Chichester (United Kingdom): Blackwell Publishing; 2011. p. 75–85.

6. Schiefelbein HM, MacLeay JM, Raymond-Loher IV, et al. Effect of diet acclimatization and length of collection on relative super saturation for calcium oxalate and struvite and the calcium oxalate risk index in cats [abstract]. J Vet Intern Med 2014;28(3):1082.

7. Lulich JP, Berent AC, Adams LG, et al. ACVIM small animal consensus recommendations on the treatment and prevention of uroliths in dogs and cats. J Vet Intern Med 2016;30(5):1564–74.

8. Buckley CM, Hawthorne A, Colyer A, et al. Effect of dietary water intake on urinary output, specific gravity and relative supersaturation for calcium oxalate and struvite in the cat. Br J Nutr 2011;106(Suppl 1):S128–30.

9. Thomas DG, Post M, Bosch G. The effect of changing the moisture levels of dry extruded and wet canned diets on physical activity in cats. J Nutr Sci 2017;6:e9.

10. Stevenson AE, Hynds WK, Markwell PJ. Effect of dietary moisture and sodium content on urine composition and calcium oxalate relative supersaturation in healthy miniature schnauzers and Labrador retrievers. Res Vet Sci 2003;74(2): 145–51.

11. Lulich JP, Osborne CA, Sanderson SL. Effects of dietary supplementation with sodium chloride on urinary relative supersaturation with calcium oxalate in healthy dogs. Am J Vet Res 2005;66(2):319–24.

12. Hawthorne AJ, Markwell PJ. Dietary sodium promotes increased water intake and urine volume in cats. J Nutr 2004;134(8 Suppl):2128S–9S.

13. Passlack N, Burmeier H, Brenten T, et al. Short term effects of increasing dietary salt concentrations on urine composition in healthy cats. Vet J 2014;201(3):401–5.

14. Queau Y, Le Verger L, Feugier A, et al. Effects of gradual increase of dietary sodium chloride on urinary parameters and relative supersaturation in healthy cats [abstract]. J Vet Intern Med 2015;29(4):1212.

15. Xu H, Laflamme DP, Bartges JW. Effect of dietary sodium on urine characteristics in healthy adult cats [abstract]. J Vet Intern Med 2006;20:738.

16. Kirk CA, Jewell DE, Lowry SR. Effects of sodium chloride on selected parameters in cats. Vet Ther 2006;7(4):333–46.

17. Reynolds BS, Chetboul V, Nguyen P, et al. Effects of dietary salt intake on renal function: a 2-year study in healthy aged cats. J Vet Intern Med 2013;27(3): 507–15.

18. Xu H, Laflamme DP, Long GL. Effects of dietary sodium chloride on health parameters in mature cats. J Feline Med Surg 2009;11(6):435–41.

19. Buranakarl C, Mathur S, Brown SA. Effects of dietary sodium chloride intake on renal function and blood pressure in cats with normal and reduced renal function. Am J Vet Res 2004;65(5):620–7.

20. Cowgill LD, Segev G, Bandt C. Effects of dietary salt intake on body fluid volume and renal function in healthy cats [abstract]. J Vet Intern Med 2007;21:600.

21. Greco DS, Lees GE, Dzendzel G, et al. Effects of dietary sodium intake on blood pressure measurements in partially nephrectomized dogs. Am J Vet Res 1994; 55(1):160–5.

22. Greco DS, Lees GE, Dzendzel GS, et al. Effect of dietary sodium intake on glomerular filtration rate in partially nephrectomized dogs. Am J Vet Res 1994; 55(1):152–9.

23. Chetboul V, Reynolds BS, Trehiou-Sechi E, et al. Cardiovascular effects of dietary salt intake in aged healthy cats: a 2-year prospective randomized, blinded, and controlled study. PLoS One 2014;9(6):e97862.

24. Xu H, Laflamme D, Bathnagar S, et al. Effect of high sodium diet on blood pressure and cardiac function in healthy adult dogs [abstract]. J Vet Intern Med 2016; 30(4):1485.

25. Pastoor FJ, Van 't Klooster AT, Opitz R, et al. Effect of dietary magnesium level on urinary and faecal excretion of calcium, magnesium and phosphorus in adult, ovariectomized cats. Br J Nutr 1995;74(1):77–84.

26. Pastoor FJ, Van 't Klooster AT, Mathot JN, et al. Increasing phosphorus intake reduces urinary concentrations of magnesium and calcium in adult ovariectomized cats fed purified diets. J Nutr 1995;125(5):1334–41.

27. Lekcharoensuk C, Osborne CA, Lulich JP, et al. Association between dietary factors and calcium oxalate and magnesium ammonium phosphate urolithiasis in cats. J Am Vet Med Assoc 2001;219(9):1228–37.

28. Finke MD, Litzenberger BA. Effect of food intake on urine pH in cats. J Small Anim Pract 1992;33:261–5.

29. Ching SV, Fettman MJ, Hamar DW, et al. The effect of chronic dietary acidification using ammonium chloride on acid-base and mineral metabolism in the adult cat. J Nutr 1989;119(6):902–15.

30. Dow SW, Fettman MJ, Smith KR, et al. Effects of dietary acidification and potassium depletion on acid-base balance, mineral metabolism and renal function in adult cats. J Nutr 1990;120(6):569–78.

31. Ching SV, Norrdin RW, Fettman MJ, et al. Trabecular bone remodeling and bone mineral density in the adult cat during chronic dietary acidification with ammonium chloride. J Bone Miner Res 1990;5(6):547–56.

32. Fettman MJ, Coble JM, Hamar DW, et al. Effect of dietary phosphoric acid supplementation on acid-base balance and mineral and bone metabolism in adult cats. Am J Vet Res 1992;53(11):2125–35.

33. Bartges JW, Kirk CA, Cox SK, et al. Influence of acidifying or alkalinizing diets on bone mineral density and urine relative supersaturation with calcium oxalate and struvite in healthy cats. Am J Vet Res 2013;74(10):1347–52.

34. Osborne CA, Lulich JP, Bartges JW, et al. Medical dissolution and prevention of canine and feline uroliths: diagnostic and therapeutic caveats. Vet Rec 1990; 127(15):369–73.

35. Houston DM, Rinkardt NE, Hilton J. Evaluation of the efficacy of a commercial diet in the dissolution of feline struvite bladder uroliths. Vet Ther 2004;5(3):187–201.

36. Houston DM, Weese HE, Evason MD, et al. A diet with a struvite relative supersaturation less than 1 is effective in dissolving struvite stones in vivo. Br J Nutr 2011; 106(Suppl 1):S90–2.

37. Lulich JP, Kruger JM, Macleay JM, et al. Efficacy of two commercially available, low-magnesium, urine-acidifying dry foods for the dissolution of struvite uroliths in cats. J Am Vet Med Assoc 2013;243(8):1147–53.

38. Torres-Henderson C, Bunkers J, Contreras ET, et al. Use of Purina Pro Plan veterinary diet UR Urinary St/Ox to dissolve struvite cystoliths. Top Companion Anim Med 2017;32(2):49–54.

39. Osborne CA, Lulich JP, Polzin DJ, et al. Medical dissolution and prevention of canine struvite urolithiasis. Twenty years of experience. Vet Clin North Am Small Anim Pract 1999;29(1):73–111, xi.

40. Rinkardt NE, Houston DM. Dissolution of infection-induced struvite bladder stones by using a noncalculolytic diet and antibiotic therapy. Can Vet J 2004; 45(10):838–40.

41. Calabro S, Tudisco R, Bianchi S, et al. Management of struvite uroliths in dogs. Br J Nutr 2011;106(Suppl 1):S191–3.

42. Lulich JP, Osborne CA, Lekcharoensuk C, et al. Effects of diet on urine composition of cats with calcium oxalate urolithiasis. J Am Anim Hosp Assoc 2004;40(3): 185–91.

43. Stevenson AE, Blackburn JM, Markwell PJ, et al. Nutrient intake and urine composition in calcium oxalate stone-forming dogs: comparison with healthy dogs and impact of dietary modification. Vet Ther 2004;5(3):218–31.

44. Pineda C, Aguilera-Tejero E, Raya AI, et al. Effects of two calculolytic diets on parameters of feline mineral metabolism. J Small Anim Pract 2015;56(8):499–504.

45. Lekcharoensuk C, Osborne CA, Lulich JP, et al. Associations between dry dietary factors and canine calcium oxalate uroliths. Am J Vet Res 2002;63(3):330–7.

46. Lekcharoensuk C, Osborne CA, Lulich JP, et al. Associations between dietary factors in canned food and formation of calcium oxalate uroliths in dogs. Am J Vet Res 2002;63(2):163–9.

47. Stevenson AE, Hynds WK, Markwell PJ. The relative effects of supplemental dietary calcium and oxalate on urine composition and calcium oxalate relative supersaturation in healthy adult dogs. Res Vet Sci 2003;75(1):33–41.

48. Dijcker JC, Hagen-Plantinga EA, Everts H, et al. Factors contributing to the variation in feline urinary oxalate excretion rate. J Anim Sci 2014;92(3):1029–36.

49. Dijcker JC, Hagen-Plantinga EA, Thomas DG, et al. The effect of dietary hydroxyproline and dietary oxalate on urinary oxalate excretion in cats. J Anim Sci 2014; 92(2):577–84.

50. von Unruh GE, Voss S, Sauerbruch T, et al. Dependence of oxalate absorption on the daily calcium intake. J Am Soc Nephrol 2004;15(6):1567–73.

51. Dijcker JC, Plantinga EA, van Baal J, et al. Influence of nutrition on feline calcium oxalate urolithiasis with emphasis on endogenous oxalate synthesis. Nutr Res Rev 2011;24(1):96–110.

52. Bai SC, Sampson DA, Morris JG, et al. Vitamin B-6 requirement of growing kittens. J Nutr 1989;119(7):1020–7.

53. Wrigglesworth DJ, Stevenson AE, Smith BH, et al. Effect of pyridoxine hydrochloride on feline urine pH and urinary relative supersaturation of calcium oxalate. [abstract]. Proceedings of the 42nd British Small Animal Veterinary Association Conference. London. 1999. p. 324.

54. Zemel MB, Schuette SA, Hegsted M, et al. Role of the sulfur-containing amino acids in protein-induced hypercalciuria in men. J Nutr 1981;111(3):545–52.

55. Hashimoto M, Funaba M, Abe M, et al. Dietary protein levels affect water intake and urinary excretion of magnesium and phosphorus in laboratory cats. Exp Anim 1995;44(1):29–35.

56. Dijcker JC, Hagen-Plantinga EA, Hendriks WH. Changes in dietary macronutrient profile do not appear to affect endogenous urinary oxalate excretion in healthy adult cats. Vet J 2012;194(2):235–9.

57. Passlack N, Kohn B, Doherr MG, et al. Influence of protein concentration and quality in a canned diet on urine composition, apparent nutrient digestibility and energy supply in adult cats. BMC Vet Res 2018;14(1):225.

58. Passlack N, Burmeier H, Brenten T, et al. Relevance of dietary protein concentration and quality as risk factors for the formation of calcium oxalate stones in cats. J Nutr Sci 2014;3:e51.

59. Kennedy SM, Lulich JP, Ritt MG, et al. Comparison of body condition score and urinalysis variables between dogs with and without calcium oxalate uroliths. J Am Vet Med Assoc 2016;249(11):1274–80.

60. Buffington CA, Rogers QR, Morris JG. Effect of diet on struvite activity product in feline urine. Am J Vet Res 1990;51(12):2025–30.

61. Queau Y, Hoek I, Feugier A, et al. Urinary pH affects urinary calcium excretion but not calcium oxalate relative supersaturation in healthy cats. J Vet Intern Med 2013;27(3):738–9.

62. Stevenson AE, Wrigglesworth DJ, Smith BH, et al. Effects of dietary potassium citrate supplementation on urine pH and urinary relative supersaturation of calcium oxalate and struvite in healthy dogs. Am J Vet Res 2000;61(4):430–5.

63. Dijcker JC, Kummeling A, Hagen-Plantinga EA, et al. Urinary oxalate and calcium excretion by dogs and cats diagnosed with calcium oxalate urolithiasis. Vet Rec 2012;171(25):646.

64. Furrow E, Patterson EE, Armstrong PJ, et al. Fasting urinary calcium-to-creatinine and oxalate-to-creatinine ratios in dogs with calcium oxalate urolithiasis and breed-matched controls. J Vet Intern Med 2015;29(1):113–9.

65. Lulich J, Kruger JM, MacLeay J, et al. A two-year-long prospective, randomized, double-masked study of nutrition on the recurrence of calcium oxalate urolithiasis in stone forming cats. Paper presented at: ACVIM Forum2014, June 4–7. Nashville, TN.

66. Allen HS, Swecker WS, Becvarova I, et al. Associations of diet and breed with recurrence of calcium oxalate cystic calculi in dogs. J Am Vet Med Assoc 2015;246(10):1098–103.

67. O'Kell AL, Grant DC, Khan SR. Pathogenesis of calcium oxalate urinary stone disease: species comparison of humans, dogs, and cats. Urolithiasis 2017;45(4):329–36.

68. Kruger JM, Osborne CA, Lulich JP. Canine calcium phosphate uroliths. Etiopathogenesis, diagnosis, and management. Vet Clin North Am Small Anim Pract 1999;29(1):141–59, xii.
69. Bartges JW, Osborne CA, Lulich JP, et al. Canine urate urolithiasis. Etiopathogenesis, diagnosis, and management. Vet Clin North Am Small Anim Pract 1999; 29(1):161–91, xii-xiii.
70. Malandain E, Causse E, Tournier C, et al. Quantification of end-products of purine catabolism in dogs fed diets varying in protein and purine content. J Vet Intern Med 2008;22(3):732–3.
71. Bartges JW, Osborne CA, Felice LJ, et al. Diet effect on activity product ratios of uric acid, sodium urate, and ammonium urate in urine formed by healthy beagles. Am J Vet Res 1995;56(3):329–33.
72. Bartges JW, Osborne CA, Felice LJ, et al. Influence of two amounts of dietary casein on uric acid, sodium urate, and ammonium urate urinary activity product ratios of healthy beagles. Am J Vet Res 1995;56(7):893–7.
73. Westropp JL, Larsen JA, Johnson EG, et al. Evaluation of dogs with genetic hyperuricosuria and urate urolithiasis consuming a purine restricted diet: a pilot study. BMC Vet Res 2017;13(1):45.
74. Lulich J, Osborne C, Bartges J, et al. Effects of diets on urate urolith recurrence in Dalmatians [abstract]. J Vet Intern Med 1997;11(2):129.
75. Bartges J, Cox S, Callens A, et al. Comparison of a soy protein hydrolysate and a low-protein diet on urinary urate saturation in dalmatians. Paper presented at: 10th Annual AAVN Clinical Nutrition & Research Symposium 2010, June 9. Anaheim, CA.
76. Hess MC, Sullivan MX. Canine cystinuria. The effect of feeding cystine, cysteine and methionine at different dietary protein levels. J Biol Chem 1942;143:545–50.
77. Osborne CA, Sanderson SL, Lulich JP, et al. Canine cystine urolithiasis. Cause, detection, treatment, and prevention. Vet Clin North Am Small Anim Pract 1999; 29(1):193–211, xiii.
78. Bartges JW, Callens AJ. Urolithiasis. Vet Clin North Am Small Anim Pract 2015; 45(4):747–68.
79. Hoppe A, Denneberg T. Cystinuria in the dog: clinical studies during 14 years of medical treatment. J Vet Intern Med 2001;15(4):361–7.
80. Sanderson SL, Osborne CA, Lulich JP, et al. Evaluation of urinary carnitine and taurine excretion in 5 cystinuric dogs with carnitine and taurine deficiency. J Vet Intern Med 2001;15(2):94–100.

Chronic Lower Urinary Tract Signs in Cats

Current Understanding of Pathophysiology and Management

Jodi L. Westropp, DVM, PhD*, Mikel Delgado, PhD, CAAB,
C. A. Tony Buffington, DVM, PhD

KEYWORDS

- Chronic lower urinary tract signs • Indoor house cats
- Multi-modal environmental modifications • Central threat response system

KEY POINTS

- Clinical research on cats with cLUTS has identified genetic factors, epigenetic influences, and environmental influences associated with cLUTS.
- Clinicians should take a "global" approach when obtaining a history, performing the physical examination, and considering pertinent diagnostics and therapeutics to manage the clinical signs of their patients.
- We currently perceive FIC to be an "anxiopathy" - pathology resulting from chronic activation of the central threat response system (CTRS).
- Early intervention with MEMO could help prevent an initial episode, or to prevent a single episode from progressing to a chronic disease.

INTRODUCTION

This article is dedicated to the memory of Dr Carl Osborne, who in 1984 suggested that, "the term feline urologic syndrome be substituted with descriptive terms pertaining to the site (urethra, bladder, and so on), causes (bacteria, parasites, neoplasms, metabolic disturbances, idiopathic forms, and so on), morphologic changes (inflammation, neoplasia, and so on), and pathophysiologic mechanisms (obstructive uropathy, reflex dyssynergia and so on) whenever possible."[1] Unfortunately this advice was not implemented, and the name feline lower urinary tract disease (FLUTD)

Funding provided for many of the studies mentioned in this article are from the NIDDK and Maddie's Fund; National Center for Advancing Translational Sciences, National Institutes of Health, through grant number UL1 TR001860 and linked award TL1 TR001861.
Department of Veterinary Medicine and Epidemiology University of California Davis, Davis, CA 95694, USA
* Corresponding author.
E-mail address: jlwestropp@ucdavis.edu

replaced feline urologic syndrome (FUS). Similar to FUS, these terms focus primarily on the lower urinary tract (LUT) system, but do not specifically define the problem.

Clinical signs referable to the LUT of indoor-housed cats have been described in the veterinary literature for nearly a century.[2] The terms FUS and FLUTD were used in the 1970s (FUS[3]) and 1980s (FLUTD[1]) to describe the variable combinations of straining, hematuria, pollakiuria (frequent passage of small amounts of urine), and periuria (urinations outside the litter box) seen in cats. In cats with acute lower urinary tract signs (LUTS), signs recur in 40% to 60% of cats,[4,5] which we define as chronic LUTS (cLUTS).

No definitive urologic explanation for these clinical signs is determined in approximately two-thirds of adult (1–10 years of age) cats with cLUTS; we refer to these patients as having feline idiopathic/interstitial cystitis (FIC). The word "interstitial" was chosen only because of the similarities between cats and humans with interstitial cystitis (now commonly referred to as bladder pain syndrome/interstitial cystitis [BPS/IC]), an idiopathic pelvic pain syndrome of human beings characterized by difficult, painful, and frequent urinations without a diagnosable cause,[6] and often a variety of other health problems.[7] The term "cystitis" is archaic[8]; no significant inflammatory response is seen in the bladder of cats with FIC.[9]

Acronyms, such as FUS or FLUTD, to describe cats with cLUTS provide only a vague description focused on the end organ, rather than a more contemporary understanding of the etiopathogenesis of most cases of cLUTS. One of the authors (C.A.T.B.) has proposed the term "Pandora syndrome" to describe the problems present in some of these cats, for at least two reasons: it does not identify any specific cause or organ; and it seems to capture the dismay and dispute associated with the identification of so many problems outside the organ of interest of any particular subspecialty.[10,11]

Clinical research on cats with cLUTS has identified genetic factors, epigenetic influences, and environmental influences associated with cLUTS[12]; documented that comorbid disorders often occur before the onset of the LUTS[13]; and demonstrated how much systemic involvement can occur in these patients.[14] Whereas invasive (and mostly ineffective) treatments for humans with BPS/IC aim at the bladder, management also is slowly evolving to treat this disorder as a systemic syndrome.[15,16] Similar to humans, evidence has accumulated that additional problems outside the LUT are commonly present in cats with cLUTS.[17] This evidence has led to reconsideration of the causes of the syndrome in these individuals, and to considerable debate about the most appropriate diagnostic and treatment recommendations. Regardless of the name used for this "syndrome," we urge clinicians to take a global approach when obtaining a history, performing the physical examination, and considering pertinent diagnostics and therapeutics to manage the clinical signs of their patients. However, to avoid confusion, we still refer to this syndrome as FIC, because it was the term used at the time many studies were published.

We currently perceive FIC to be an anxiopathy, pathology resulting from chronic activation of the central threat response system (CTRS).[10] Persistent activation of this system by the presence of chronic perception of threat that exceeds the cat's perception of control mobilizes activity in variable combinations of the nervous (sensory, autonomic, and motor), endocrine, and immune systems, which can eventually result in pathology affecting any combination of organ systems.[18]

The variability in response to chronic perception of threat may result from familial differences in organ-specific vulnerability, and to the intensity of exposure to threatening events that can durably sensitize the CTRS to the environment. Such events often occur early in life, even before birth, when the CTRS is most plastic and vulnerable to the events communicated to it through the placenta by its mother.[12] Sufficiently harsh events can sensitize the CTRS at any time of life, however.

HISTOPATHOLOGY AND BIOMARKERS

Two forms of BPS/IC are recognized in humans, the common (>90% of cases) non-ulcerative (type I) and uncommon (<10%) Hunner ulcer ulcerative form (type II).[19] Most cats with FIC have signs comparable with the type I form, although the type II form has been described in a cat.[20] It is possible that the etiopathogenesis of these two forms is different in cats, as it seems to be in humans. Type II seems to include a conventional inflammatory response, whereas type I might be more associated with neuroendocrine-immune abnormalities (see later). No well-accepted diagnostic test for FIC currently exists, although research evaluating urine and serum biomarkers has been published (none of these biomarkers are currently available).[21–23] Recently, various proinflammatory cytokines and chemokines (eg, CXCL12, interleukin-12, interleukin-18, and FLT3L)[24] were noted to be increased in the serum of cats with FIC. Cystoscopy and biopsies were not obtained in that study to document if any characteristic ulcerative or other inflammatory lesions were present in those cats. Moreover, no evidence permits one to discriminate between these changes being antecedents, consequences, or differences not directly related to the problem. Given other evidence of the success of various therapeutic approaches (discussed later), it seems that these changes may be a consequence of some underlying disorder.

RESEARCH ON FELINE IDIOPATHIC/INTERSTITIAL CYSTITIS: BLADDER AND BEYOND

Bladder epithelial, called urothelial, cells can respond to various stimuli, including adenosine triphosphate and nitric oxide, which could potentiate inflammation and exacerbate clinical signs in cats with FIC.[25] The bladder (and nonbladder) sensory neurons in cats with FIC exhibit an increased excitability to physical and chemical stimuli as compared with unaffected cats, albeit outside the normal range of bladder pressure.[26]

Sympathoneural-epithelial interactions also seem to play an important role in the permeability of the urothelium. Birder and colleagues[27] have shown that application of norepinephrine to urinary bladder strips induced the release of nitric oxide from the urothelium. Application of capsaicin, the active compound in hot peppers, also resulted in the release of nitric oxide from urothelium, and nervous tissue in the urinary bladder. In light of reports that nitric oxide may increase permeability in the urothelium[28] (and elsewhere),[29,30] these results suggest that some of the sympathetically mediated alterations in permeability may be mediated by norepinephrine via this mechanism.

In humans presenting with cLUTS, urodynamic evaluations are often performed to rule out other LUT diseases, such as overactive bladder (OAB), which could account for the clinical signs. Urodynamic studies in humans have found that patients with BPS/IC had fewer episodes of urge incontinence and shorter duration of symptoms compared with those with OAB.[31] Furthermore they had significantly decreased maximal bladder capacity compared with women with OAB. Although a decrease in bladder compliance has been found in cats with FIC, no evidence of spontaneous bladder contractions (OAB) was noted in female cats with FIC when cystometrograms were evaluated.[32] However, increased urethral closure pressures were noted in cats with FIC compared with healthy cats, despite a lack of clinical signs at the time the studies were performed.

Clinical signs of FIC can wax and wane, and seem to be exacerbated by internal and external stressors.[33] Elevations in catecholamine and decreases in serum cortisol concentrations in cats with FIC compared with healthy cats during times of acute and chronic stress have been reported, suggesting an uncoupling of these two parameters of the stress response. Based on this research, we believe that FIC may include multiple, complex, and variable abnormalities of the nervous, endocrine, and immune systems that likely affect more than just the bladder.[11,34–36] Enhanced central noradrenergic drive in the face of inadequate adrenocortical restraint seems to be related to maintaining the chronic disease process. These systems seem to be driven by tonically increased hypothalamic corticotropin-releasing factor release, which may represent the outcome of a developmental accident.[37] Treatment strategies that decrease the activity of the CTRS seem to reduce signs of FIC; those that do not address this aspect of the disease seem to be less effective. Until more effective treatments to normalize the responsiveness of this system are available, efforts to reduce input to this system by effective multimodal environmental modification (MEMO) has been shown to effectively reduce clinical signs of FIC and related comorbidities in affected cats (discussed later).[36,38]

It has also become apparent that humans with BPS/IC often overlap or share symptoms commonly associated with other persistent pain disorders, such as irritable bowel syndrome and fibromyalgia, and even OAB.[16] Similarly, cats can present with other comorbidities in addition to the LUTS. A study of healthy cats and cats with FIC found that environmental stressors resulted in increased number of sickness behaviors (eg, vomiting, lethargy, and anorexia) in cats with FIC when the results were controlled for other factors.[36] Furthermore, cats with FIC have a variable combination of comorbid disorders,[17,39,40] such as behavioral, endocrine, cardiovascular, and gastrointestinal problems. Therefore, a complete physical examination and detailed environmental history must be obtained from owners of these cats, rather than restricting focus entirely on the bladder, to appreciate the complexity of some cases.

RECENT EPIDEMIOLOGIC STUDIES

Lund and colleagues[41] recently reported that obesity ($P = .004$), nervous disposition ($P = .007$), and frequent diet changes ($P = .025$) were found significantly more often in 70 cats with FIC in the final multivariate model of their matched, case-control study when compared with 95 control cats in Norway. Defauw and colleagues,[42] using a retrospective, case-controlled design, found similar results, and also reported that inactive lifestyle and increased threat responsiveness were significantly (all P values < 0.01) more commonly found in 64 cats with FIC than in 64 control cats in Belgium. A more recent case-controlled study of 58 cats with FIC and 281 randomly selected control cats living in a primarily indoor environment in South Korea found that cats with FIC were 2.53 times (odds ratio; $P = .006$) more likely to live in an apartment than in a house, 2.62 times ($P = .003$) more likely to have access only to nonclumping litter, 3.16 times ($P = .001$) more likely to live with other cats, and 4.64 times ($P<.001$) more likely *not* to have a vantage point they could climb on.[43] Although urethral obstruction occurs more commonly in male than in female cats, this is likely caused by differences in the anatomy of the urethra. Underlying FIC is thought to be the cause of urethral obstruction in some, perhaps many, cases.[44] Moreover, the epidemiology of the urethral obstruction in male cats seems broadly similar to that found in most epidemiologic studies of FIC.[45]

All of these studies provide additional evidence for the presence of complex interactions between susceptible individuals and provocative environments in the development of cLUTS.[33] Knowing these risk factors can help clinicians tailor treatment protocols to the cat's environmental circumstances (see later) or better yet, optimize the environment early in the cat's life to help prevent cLUTS associated with FIC.

Moreover, effective environmental management is an essential part of the responsibility to protect the health and welfare of confined animals (https://www.avma.org/KB/Resources/Reference/AnimalWelfare/Pages/default.aspx. Accessed January 8, 2019).[46]

DIAGNOSTIC EVALUATION OF CATS WITH LOWER URINARY TRACT SIGNS

When choosing the appropriate diagnostic tests for a cat that is presented for evaluation of LUTS, several factors need to be taken into consideration, including the number of episodes the cat has had, the severity of the cat's clinical signs, and the financial limitations of the owner. Because no sensitive, specific, and clinically available test currently exists to diagnose FIC, the diagnosis rests on signalment, history, including inclusion of cat and environmental risk factors as described previously, exclusion of other (common) causes of LUTS, and response to therapy (see **algorithm**).

Most adult middle-aged cats with cLUTS are eventually diagnosed with FIC, so we often begin by offering treatment of FIC and monitoring the cat's response, watching carefully for a positive response, particularly if the owner has financial constraints and declines additional diagnostic testing (eg, urinalysis, imaging). If the cat does not improve, or if clinical signs return within days to weeks despite implementation of appropriate MEMO, we recommend abdominal radiography because the next most common differential in cats with cLUTS is urinary stone disease. Abdominal radiography, including the entire urinary system from the proximal pole of the kidney to beyond the end of the distal urethra, helps detect radiodense stones; approximately 20% of cats with LUTS have bladder stones. A urinalysis and urine bacterial culture should be evaluated at least once in cats with cLUTS if possible, but most young, otherwise healthy cats do not have a true bacterial cystitis. Furthermore, there is no sound evidence to support culture of the urine after urinary catheter removal from cats with obstructive FIC unless clinical signs have returned or progressed.

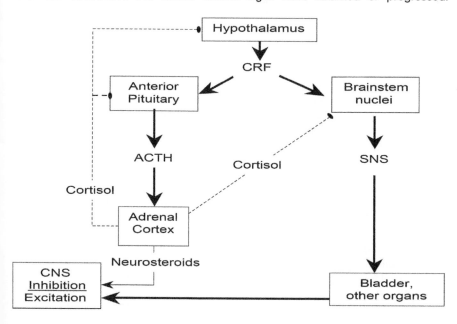

Antimicrobial therapy is not recommended unless the cat has LUTS in association with a positive urine culture collected by cystocentesis. Advanced diagnostic tests, such as contrast cystourethrography, abdominal ultrasonography, and even cystoscopy, are performed in recurrent cases to be certain no other disease that could account for the clinical signs is present. The latter is rarely required or performed in cats suspected of having FIC.

TREATMENT OF CATS WITH CHRONIC LOWER URINARY TRACT SIGNS
Acute Treatment

LUTS resolve in 85% of cats within 2 to 7 days, with or without treatment. Most aspects of acute therapy have not been adequately tested to permit evidence-based recommendations. Because of the presumed threat sensitivity of cats with FIC, we try to use pertinent trauma-informed care principles with clients and their cats (eg, safety, predictability, empowerment, choice, shared decision making).[47] Low-stress handling techniques and predictable nursing care can reduce cats' perception of threat.[35,48] If the patient is hospitalized, careful consideration of the quality of the cage environment may help the cat cope with this confinement.[48,49] Cats tend to form attachments to places, so confinement in places where they do not feel safe can adversely affect their behavior and physiology. Enriched conditions permit cats to cope with their surroundings and feel more safe in their space.

Factors inside and outside their cage can affect the welfare of cats housed in veterinary hospitals.[35] Inside the cage, each cat needs these resources at its disposal:

- A place to hide: Cats like places to hide to escape threats, keep warm, and to scratch and perch on. We place these at the back of the cage to try to help the cat feel safer.
- Bedding: Cover the bottom of the cage completely. Bare surfaces can be cold and uncomfortable. Bedding with the cat's and owner's scent also may reduce cats' perception of threat. Change bedding only when soiled (rather than daily); most cats seem to prefer familiar bedding.
- Food and water: Provide the cat's usual food if feasible, and put food and water at the back of the cage as close as possible to its hiding place to help the cat feel safer.
- Litter box: Place at the front of the cage, because cats use it less frequently than (and only after) they use eating and drinking bowls.
- Other things: Provide music (played softly), and extra attention like brushing or playing from a familiar, dedicated person whenever possible.
- Door: Cover as much of the door of the cage as possible to reduce potentially threatening stimulation.

Factors outside the cage also are stressful for confined cats.[48] These can include the following:[50]

- Lights: Put on a timer for predictable lighting from day to day if natural light is not available, or turn lights on and off manually at the same time each day. Do NOT turn lights on and off each time someone goes in and out of the ward/room.
- Noise: Keep levels in the ward to a minimum (<60 dB, a quiet conversational level, can be measured with smartphone apps).
- Odors: Minimize smells from dogs, other cats, perfumes, alcohol (from hand rubs), cigarettes, cleaning chemicals (including laundry detergent); all these are aversive and stressful, especially to cats confined in a cage where they cannot move away from the odors.

- Temperature: Cats prefer warm, 85°F to 100°F, temperatures.[51] Provide bedding that allows cats cocoon to retain warmth if they choose to do so.
- Daily routine: To the extent possible, perform cleaning, feeding, and treatment procedures at the same time each day, preferably by the same person to increase predictability of the environment for the cat. Return cage furnishings to the same place after spot-cleaning, and house cats in the same cage throughout their stay.
- Low stress handling: Use these techniques to minimize activation of the cat's CTRS.

Behaviors signaling that something may be wrong with caged cats include resting in litter boxes, and cages that show no use since the last cleaning or are in disarray. Sickness behaviors also are cause for concern.[36] These include variable combinations of vomiting, diarrhea or soft feces, no eliminations in 24 hours, urinating or defecating out of the litter box, anorexia or decreased appetite, lethargy, and not grooming.[36]

One can recognize when a cat feels threatened by observing changes in its physiology and behavior, recognizing that the changes in any one cat might be different from those of another that feels similarly threatened. Any effectiveness of any housing situation or handling technique is evaluated by assessing physiologic and behavioral parameters in the cat before and after it is applied. Physiologic and behavioral parameters associated with perception of threat include variable combinations of the following; their converse suggest perception of safety:

Physiologic parameters	
Increase in	**Presence of**
• Pupil diameter	• "Sweaty" paws
• Respiratory rate	• Excessive shedding
• Temperature	• Flushing of the skin
• Heart rate	• Anxious lip-licking
• Blood pressure	

Behavioral parameters/body postures	
Increases in withdrawal behaviors	**Decreases in affiliative ("approach") behaviors**
• Immobility: hiding, cowering, or freezing behaviors	• Friendly approach to caregivers
• Attempts to run away or avoid handlers	• Purring, kneading, rubbing
• Defensive aggression (hissing, growling, spitting, tail twitching, ear flicking, scratching, biting)	• Interest in food
	• Relaxed body postures, normal eliminations
	• Increased effectiveness of the technique with repeated use

Acute Pharmacotherapy

Analgesic therapy for acute pain management is provided when clinically indicated, which seems prudent given the clinical manifestations in cats and the pain described in humans with the syndrome. Use of nonsteroidal anti-inflammatory drugs has been suggested, but with disappointing results, at least in obstructive FIC.[52] Because of the risk for dehydration-associated reductions in blood flow to the kidneys and the potential for acute kidney injury, these medications might increase the risk for adverse outcomes. Moreover, nonsteroidal anti-inflammatory drugs have been found to be ineffective for pain management of patients with BPS/IC, and are not part of contemporary therapeutic guidelines for patients with this syndrome.[6,53] Other analgesics also have been used, but not yet been subjected to properly controlled clinical trials to our knowledge.

CHRONIC TREATMENT
Treating the Client

A diagnosis of FIC means that one has identified an anxiopathy and excluded (to the extent possible) other causes for the signs. In our experience, the most important consideration for a successful outcome for cats with FIC is effective and empathic client communication.[54] After performing a complete evaluation of the cat and concluding that FIC is likely to be present (pending observation of responsiveness to MEMO), we can explain to the client that although no cure currently is available, appropriate MEMO and other therapeutic interventions can generally keep the cat's clinical signs to a minimum and increase the disease-free interval, and that most care can be provided in collaboration with a trained technician. We also demonstrate empathy by listening carefully to the client's (often frustrated) story of the effects of having a cat with FIC, provide a satisfactory explanation for the sources of the signs, express care and concern for the situation, and enhance the client's perception of control. Effective doctor-patient interactions seem to enhance patient adherence to treatments, and quality of life outcomes of therapy.[55] We can then prescribe any therapies appropriate to the presenting manifestations, and when possible introduce the client to the technician or other staff member trained to care for cats with FIC, who coach the client to implement MEMO for the patient. The formality of this introduction demonstrates that we intend to sustain the partnership with the client through our technical support staff to gain control of the patient's clinical signs.

Treating the Environment: Multimodal Environmental Modification

Environmental conditions are known to affect the behavior and health of animals,[56,57] particularly captive animals.[50,58,59] Just as water is primary therapy for prevention of urinary stone recurrence,[60] MEMO is primary therapy for prevention of recurrence of signs of FIC. Effective MEMO has been shown to provide relief in a variety of animal models of chronic pain.[18,57,61] If cats with FIC have a sensitized CTRS, then treatments that increase their perception of control and reduce their perception of threat are more likely to be effective than those that do not. Effective MEMO creates conditions that permit the patient to feel safe, and to have unrestricted access to species-appropriate novelty, activity, and interactions with other animals (including humans). Effective MEMO for cats means provision of all necessary resources, refinement of interactions with owners, a tolerable intensity of conflict, and thoughtful institution of changes to the cat's environment (its territory). It also extends the "one + one" rule traditionally applied to litter boxes (one for each cat in the home, plus one more) to all pertinent resources (particularly resting areas, and food, water, and litter containers) in the home.

This opinion is based on the documented neuroendocrine abnormalities suffered by cats with FIC,[23,34,62] and on our research and clinical experience. Although we are not aware that a particular resource list has been validated for indoor-housed cats, some recommendations are available. We have assembled a provisional list in **Box 1** that might be used to guide consideration of these parameters for each of their cats. The following tentative recommendations are organized to follow the table; other

> **Box 1**
> **A checklist of confined cats' needs**
>
> • Safe places to rest and sleep, preferably including a carrier as one option.
>
> • An environment that accommodates all sensory modalities, including gustatory, visual, auditory, tactile, and olfactory.
>
> • Satisfactory foods, which accommodate the preferences of the owner and the cat.
>
> • Daily opportunities for the cat to play and engage in predatory behavior.
>
> • Multiple and separated areas in multicat households for key environmental resources (resting and sleeping, food, water, toileting, scratching, climbing, and play).
>
> • Changes in environmental resources offered as choices to allow the cat to express its preferences.
>
> • As positive, consistent, and predictable an environment as possible.
>
> • Positive, consistent, and predictable daily human-cat social interaction.

environmental questionnaires and suggestions are available in the many excellent publications about cat housing and behavior that currently are available.[63,64]

A prospective observational study that evaluated client-reported recurrence rates of LUTS (and other behavioral problems) in cats with FIC after MEMO therapy suggested that this form of therapy is beneficial for cats with FIC. Clients were asked to complete a detailed environmental history sheet (a similar one is found in **Fig. 1**), and specific recommendations for MEMO based on this assessment were made for each client.[38] Cases were followed for 10 months, primarily by telephone contact. Significant ($P<.05$) reductions in LUTS, fearfulness, nervousness, signs referable to the respiratory tract, and a trend ($P<.1$) toward reduced aggressive behavior and signs referable to the lower intestinal tract were identified. Additionally, experimental studies of rodents subjected to early adverse experience have documented psychoneuroendocrine abnormalities, which may be compensated for, if not repaired by, MEMO.[65–67] Not all cats require intense MEMO therapy, so clinicians can tailor the MEMO changes implemented based on the cats' needs and owner's desire and commitment to this process. Because of the lack of controlled trials, it currently is not possible to prioritize the importance of any of these suggestions provided, or to predict which would be most appropriate in any particular situation. Appropriately designed epidemiologic studies might be able to identify particularly important factors (discussed previously), after which intervention trials could be conducted to determine their effectiveness in circumstances where owners successfully implemented the suggested changes.

Space

Provide safe resting places for each cat. Using an inviting soft fabric or hard plastic cat carrier for one of these places also helps habituate the cat to its carrier and can facilitate transport when necessary. Some cats also enjoy using beds heated with warming pads made specifically for pet beds. Cats interact with the physical structures and other animals, including humans, in their environment. The physical environment should include opportunities for scratching (horizontal and vertical may be necessary), climbing, and hiding in addition to resting. Cats seem to prefer to monitor their surroundings from elevated vantage points, so climbing frames, hammocks, platforms, raised walkways, shelves, or window seats may appeal to them. Playing a sound source to habituate cats to sudden changes in sound and human voices in their

Health History Questionnaire – (one for each cat)

Your Last Name:_____ This cat's name:_____

Your ZIP code:_____ Today's Date: _____

Description: Breed:_____ Color:_____ Birthdate _____ Weight:_____ ☐ lb. ☐kg

Owned for: _____ years; ☐ Male ☐Female Neutered? ☐ No ☐Yes if yes, Date:_____

Declawed? ☐N   ☐Y   If yes, Front paws only ☐   All four paws ☐

Body Condition (please check box that looks most like this cat):

☐Skinny	☐Lean	☐Moderate	☐Stout	☐Obese

Diet: please include the name of the food, the company that makes it, and the flavor of the food

Food:	% of TOTAL daily food eaten by this cat
Wet: _____	☐None ☐25% ☐50% ☐75% ☐100%
Dry: _____	☐None ☐25% ☐50% ☐75% ☐100%
Other: _____	☐None ☐25% ☐50% ☐75% ☐100%

Where did you get this cat?
☐Offspring from a pet I already own(ed)   ☐From a shelter/rescue organization
☐From a friend   ☐Stray/orphan
☐From a breeder   ☐Gift
☐From a pet shop   ☐Other (please describe)

How many hours a day, on average, does this cat spend Indoors?	☐24 - indoor Only	☐18-24	☐12-18	☐6-12	☐0-6
Is time outside supervised?	☐Not applicable		☐Yes	☐No	

We live in: ☐ Apartment or condominium building ☐ Standalone home
☐ **Other** (please describe) _____
Total Number of Cats_____ Dogs_____ Other Pets_____ People_____ in your home

If you have more than one cat, are they related?   ☐ **No**
Yes: ☐Littermate ☐ Sibling ☐Parent-Offspring ☐Other _____

How many **hours** each day are you in sight of this cat?	_____ hours/day.
How many **minutes** each day do you pet/hold/sit near to this cat?	_____ minutes/day.
How many **minutes** each day do you spend playing with this cat?	_____ minutes/day.

Fig. 1. Environmental survey for indoor-housed cats.[1] Female pronouns are used in honor of Bastet, the Egyptian cat goddess revered for her hunting prowess and motherly nurturing skills. We love male cats too, and everything also applies to them.

surroundings also has been recommended, and videos to provide visual stimulation are available.

Food

As a part of the MEMO therapy, dietary modifications may be warranted and should be discussed with clients. Efforts to acidify the urine using dry foods have no proven value in the treatment of cats with FIC; however, if pronounced struvite crystalluria is present in an obstructed male cat (ie, obstructive FIC), a diet formulated to produce a urinary pH less than the relative supersaturation for struvite may be indicated. A diet high in moisture (eg, canned food) also may help prevent recurrences, but studies to evaluate

What Does Your Cat Do

Thinking about the **last 4 weeks** My cat:	Almost always	Repeatedly	Often	Some times	Seldom	Rarely	Never
1 Moves around our home free to explore, climb, stretch, or play as she[1] chooses.							
2 Approaches people to be sociable.							
3 Avoids being held, picked up, handled or petted.							
4 Actively plays with toys, others, or self.							
5 Uses a climbing tree/elevated vantage point to rest or have an overview of her surroundings.							
6 Is easily startled.							
7 Uses an "approved" object to scratch on.							
8 Remains calm when left alone.							
9 Eats and drinks small amounts calmly often throughout the 24-hour day.							
10 Tries to escape to the outdoors.							
11 Cries or paces at doors to the outside.							
12 Chase or attacks people's hands, feet, or ankles.							
13 Chase or attacks other animals.							
14 Lies on side while relaxing.							
15 Growls, hisses, bites or scratches when approached.							
16 Makes positive sounds, like purring, chirping or friendly meowing.							

	Almost always	Repeatedly	Often	Some times	Seldom	Rarely	Never
17 I correct/punish this cat for behaviors that annoy me							
18 **Our home** is quiet.							
19 **Our household schedule** is predictable from day to day.							

[1] I use female pronouns in honor of Bastet, the Egyptian cat goddess revered both for her hunting prowess *and* motherly nurturing skills. We love male cats too, and everything also applies to them.

Fig. 1. (*continued*).

this effect have not been conclusive to date. Although we have demonstrated that feeding wet food is not essential in enriched environments,[36,38] it may be more beneficial in environments that are less enriched, although to our knowledge this has not been studied in a controlled trial. Cats may find wet food to be preferable because of the increased water content, or to a more natural "mouth feel," whereas some cats seem to strongly to prefer dry foods. Obesity often is associated with FIC, so implementing a MEMO-based weight loss program also may be of benefit, if clinically indicated, but should be approached cautiously to avoid overwhelming the client with recommendations.[68]

Your Cat's Environment – (one for each household, or each cat if different)

We ask the following questions to get a better idea of your home from your cat's point of view. In homes with more than one cat, some cats like to have their "stuff" (resting area, food and water, litter box, etc.) **out of sight of all other cat's stuff**, so think about where each cat's stuff is if you have more than one cat as you fill out the form.

#	Space	Yes	No
1	Each cat has a personal space that provides her with safety and security.		
2	Each personal space is located such that another animal or person cannot sneak up on your cat(s) while they are resting.		
3	Each personal space is located away from appliances or air ducts that could come on unexpectedly while your cat(s) are resting.		
4	Scented candles, incense, perfume or other fragrances are commonly used in our home.		
5	There are sights (like other animals), sounds (like construction or traffic) or smells (like other animals) outside our home that might disturb our cat(s).		
#	Food and Water	Yes	No
6	Each cat has her own food bowl.		
7	Each cat has her own water bowl.		
8	Both food and water bowls are located out of sight of all other cat's bowls.		
9	Both food and water bowls are located at least 3 feet (1 meter) from the nearest litter box.		
10	All bowls are located such that another animal or person cannot sneak up on each cat while she eats or drinks.		
11	All bowls are located away from appliances or air ducts that could come on unexpectedly while any cat is eating.		
12	Do you provide any food in food puzzles?		
#	Litter boxes	Yes	No
13	There is at least 1 box per cat + 1 extra in our home.		
14	Each cat's box is located in a convenient, well-ventilated place that still gives her some privacy while using it.		
15	Boxes are located so another animal or human cannot sneak up on each cat during use.		
16	Boxes are located away from appliances or air ducts that could come on unexpectedly during use.		
17	Boxes are as long as each cat's body, from the tip of the nose to the tip of the tail.		
18	Some boxes are covered.		
19	Unscented, clumping litter is used.		
20	There is at least enough litter in each box so each cat can scratch around without hitting bottom.		
21	Each litter box is scooped as soon after use as possible, or at least daily.		

Please write additional comments on or questions about any of the items in this form below, including the question #. _____

_____

_____

Fig. 1. (*continued*).

Diets containing additives that purportedly decrease anxiety (eg, α-casozepine and L-tryptophan) in stressed cats and those tailored for FIC management also are marketed for cats, but the evidence for their effectiveness in management of FIC have not been well investigated, and their general salutary effects, if any, seem modest.[69,70] Moreover, studies have shown that many cats with FIC are effectively managed without any diet change.[36,38,71] In most cases we recommend that clients choose whichever (Association of American Feed Control Officials labeled) diets fit their personal preferences, and then offer a few examples of these at mealtime so their cat can express its preferences. We recommend this to minimize the effects of client's and patient's perception of diet on the activation of their CTRS.

If a diet change is appropriate, offering the new diet in a separate, adjacent container rather than removing the usual food and replacing it with the new food

Your Cat's Health

Directions: Please use the following choices to describe how often this cat has done each item, both in the past years, **and** in the last 4 weeks.

In the PAST, how often has this cat: Score: 0=never, 1=at least once, 2=at least yearly, 3=a few times a year, 4=at least monthly	Score	In the LAST 4 WEEKS, how often has this cat:
Wheezed		
Sneezed		
Had discharge from nose nose		
Had discharge from eyes		
Had difficulty breathing		
Eaten more or less than usual		
Vomited ☐food ☐hair ☐bile ☐other		
Had diarrhea		
Had constipation		
Defecated outside the litter box		
Urinated outside the litter box		
Sprayed urine		
Groomed more than cats usually do		
Shed more than cats usually do		
Howled more than cats usually do		
Scratched herself more than cats usually do		

Please check any of the following diseases your veterinarian has diagnosed in this cat, and the date of diagnosis:

Disease	Date	Disease	Date
☐ Periodontal (dental) disease		☐ Asthma	
☐ Inflammatory bowel disease		☐ Chronic skin disease	
☐ Allergies		☐ Diabetes mellitus	
☐ Cardiomyopathy (heart problems)		☐ Obesity	
☐ Chronic dental disease		☐ Respiratory tract infections	
☐ Chronic kidney disease		☐ Urinary stone disease	
☐ Other_____			

Please provide any additional comments about this cat's health below:

_____

_____

_____

_____

_____

_____

Fig. 1. (*continued*).

permits the cat to express its preference. All the cat's needs must be taken into consideration when making dietary and environmental recommendations.

Behavioral and ethological research suggest that cats prefer to eat individually in a quiet location where they are not startled by other animals, sudden movement, or activity of an air duct or appliance that may begin operation unexpectedly.[72,73] Natural feline feeding behavior also includes predatory activities, such as stalking and pouncing. These may be simulated by hiding small amounts of food around the house, or by putting dry food in a food puzzle from which the cat has to extract individual pieces or move to release the food pieces (if such interventions appeal to the cat).[74] When a diet change seems appropriate, we only attempt to implement it after the cat has returned home and is feeling better to reduce the risk of inducing a learned aversion to the new food.

Water

Some cats also seem to have preferences for water that can be investigated. Water-related factors to consider include freshness, taste, movement (water fountains, dripping faucets, or aquarium pump-bubbled air into a bowl), and shape of container (some cats seem to resent having their vibrissae touch the sides of the container when drinking). As with foods, changes in water-related factors should be offered in such a way that permits the cat to express its preferences. Additionally, food and water bowls should be cleaned regularly unless individual preference suggests otherwise.

Play

Some cats seem to prefer to be petted and groomed, whereas others may prefer play interactions with owners.[75] Cats also are easily trained to perform behaviors (tricks); owners just need to understand that cats respond much better to praise than to force, and seem to be more amenable to learning if the behavior is shaped before feeding. Cats also may enjoy playing with toys, particularly those that are small, move, and that mimic prey characteristics. Many cats also prefer novelty, so a variety of toys should be provided, and rotated or replaced regularly to sustain their interest.

Some cats also seem to have specific prey preferences. For example, some cats prefer to chase birds, whereas others may prefer to chase mice or bugs. Identifying a cat's prey preference allows one to buy or make toys that the cat is more likely to play with. Prey preference are identified by paying close attention to the cat's reaction to toys with specific qualities, such as those that resemble birds (feather toys), small mammals (furry mice), or insects (laser pointers, pieces of dry food) presented one at a time or together.

Litter Boxes

Litter boxes should be provided in different locations throughout the house to the extent possible, particularly in multiple cat households.[76] Placing litter boxes in quiet, convenient locations that provide an escape route if necessary for the cat could help improve conditions for normal elimination behaviors. If different litters are offered, it may be preferable to test the cat's preferences by providing them in separate boxes, because individual preferences for litter type have been documented. For cats with a history of urinary problems, unscented clumping litter may be preferred.[77] Litter boxes should be cleaned regularly and replaced; some cats seem sensitive to dirty litter boxes. Litter box size and whether or not it is open or covered also may be important to some cats.[78,79]

Conflict

Conflict can develop between cats, and between cats and other animals and people in the home.[80] When cats become threatened, they seem to respond in an attempt to restore their perception of control. During such responses, some cats become aggressive, some become withdrawn, and some become ill. In our experience, conflict is the most common reason that some health problems occur in households with multiple cats confined indoors. With a little practice, one can recognize the signs of conflict and estimate its potential role in exacerbation of signs of FIC. Owners usually can identify the causes after the signs of conflict are explained to them. Once this has been done, clients often are well on their way to reducing the intensity of conflict.

Of course, some conflict between housemates is normal, regardless of species. The goal is to reduce unhealthy conflict to a more manageable level for the cats involved.

Signs of conflict (**Table 1**) between cats are open or silent. Signs of open conflict are easy to recognize; the cats may stalk each other, hiss, and turn sideways with legs straight and hair standing on end up to make themselves look larger. If neither cat backs down, the displays may increase to swatting, wrestling, and biting. The signs of silent conflict are so subtle they are easily missed or ignored by owners. The cat creating the conflict (assertive cat) is identified as the one that never backs away from other (threatened) cats, denies other cats' access to resources, stares at other cats, and lowers its head and neck while elevating its hindquarters as it approaches less confident cats. The hair along its back, on its tail, and tail base may stand on end, although not to the extent of cats engaged in open conflict, and it may emit a low growl. The assertive cat eventually may only have to approach or stare at a threatened cat for it to leave a resource, such as food or a litter box. If the threatened cat tries to use the resource later, the assertive cat's presence alone may be enough to make it flee. Because cats do not seem to possess distinct dominance hierarchies or conflict resolution strategies, threatened cats may attempt to circumvent agonistic encounters by avoiding other cats, by decreasing their activity, or both. Threatened cats often spend increasingly large amounts of time away from the family, staying in areas of the house that others do not use, or they attempt to interact with family members only when the assertive cat is elsewhere.

The signs of conflict can result from two types of conflict: offensive and defensive. In offensive conflict, the assertive cat moves closer to the other cats, and to control the interaction. In defensive conflict situations, a threatened cat attempts to increase the distance between itself and whatever it perceives to be a threat. Although cats engaged in either type of conflict may spray or eliminate outside the litter box, we find that threatened cats are more likely to develop FIC.

The most common cause of conflict between indoor-housed cats that we identify is competition for resources. Cats may engage in open or silent conflict over space, food, water, litter boxes, perches, sunny areas, safe places where the cat can watch its environment, or attention from people. There may be no obvious limitation to access to

Table 1	
Signs of silent conflict between cats	
The Assertive Cat	*The Threatened Cat*
Never backs away from other cats	Spends large amounts of time hiding or away from the family
Stares at other cats	Avoids eye contact with other cats
Denies other cats access resources	Yields resources to other cats
Rub cheeks, head, chin, and tail on people, doorways, and furniture at cat height	
When it sees the threatened cat	*When it sees the assertive cat*
Lowers its head and neck while elevating its hindquarters and stalks the other cat	Crouches, may cower, may then flee
Piloerects the hair along its back, tail base, and tail	
Growls	Does not vocalize
May spray	May spray
	May develop cystitis or other disease problem

these resources for conflict to develop. The change may only be the cat's perceptions of how much control it wants over the environment or its housemates' behaviors.

Open conflict is most likely to occur when a new cat is introduced into the house, and when cats that have known each other since kittenhood reach social maturity. Conflict occurring when a new cat is introduced is easy to understand, and good directions are available from many sources for introducing the new cat to the current residents.[81] Clients may be puzzled by conflict that starts when one of their cats becomes socially mature, or when a socially mature cat perceives that one of its housemates is becoming socially mature. Cats become socially mature between 2 and 5 years of age, and may start to take some control of the social groups and their activities. These actions can lead to open conflict between males, between females, or between males and females. Although clients may be surprised, "because they lived so well together for the first few years of their lives!," cat's perceptions of resource needs may expand with social maturity.

Cats that are familiar with each other but unevenly matched often show conflict in more subtle ways. One of the cats in the conflict asserts itself, and another cat is threatened by this cat's actions. Silent conflicts may not even be recognized until the threatened cat begins to hide from the assertive cat, to hiss or fight back when it sees the other cat, or when it develops a health problem.

In addition to the signs of conflict described previously, the assertive cat is identified by its marking behavior. These cats rub their cheeks, head, chin, and tail on people, doorways, and furniture at cat height. Unfortunately, silent conflict can also involve urine; including marking by the assertive or the threatened cat, and FIC in the threatened cat. Conflict-related urine marking can include spraying, when the cat treads and kneads, raises its tail, and flicks the tip of it while spraying urine on a vertical surface or squatting and urinating outside the litter box (nonspray marking). Both males and females may spray, and although neutering reduces the frequency of spraying, it cannot eliminate the behavior. Conflict-related urine marking is exhibited by either the assertive or threatened cat, but in our experience, FIC usually occurs in the threatened cat; we have even seen threatened male cats spray bloody urine. Cats that urinate on bedspreads or other elevated, open places may do so because their access to the litter box is restricted by another cat, or if they are afraid to use the box because it is placed such that a quick escape from another cat might not be possible.[64]

Treatment of conflict between cats involves providing a separate set of resources for each cat, preferably in locations where the cats can use them without being seen by other cats. This lets the cats avoid each other if they choose to without being deprived of an essential resource. Conflict also is reduced by neutering all of the cats, and by keeping all nails trimmed as short as practicable. Whenever the cats involved in the conflict cannot be directly supervised, they may need to be separated. This may mean that some of the cats in the household can stay together, but that the threatened cat is provided a refuge from the other cats. This room should contain all necessary resources for the cat staying in it. In severe cases, one or more of the cats may need to be rehomed to avoid euthanasia.

Cats in nature use more space than the average house or apartment affords them. The addition of elevated spaces, such as shelves, "kitty condos," cardboard boxes, beds, or crates may provide enough space to reduce conflict to a tolerable level. In severe situations, some cats may benefit from behavior-modifying medications. In our experience, however, medication can help only after environmental enrichment has occurred, it cannot replace it.

The cats involved in the conflict may never be "best friends," but they usually can live together without showing signs of conflict or conflict-related disease. In severe cases, a behaviorist may be consulted for assistance in desensitizing and countercon-ditioning of cats in conflict so they can share the same spaces more comfortably if this is desired.

Conflict with other animals, dogs, children, or adults is straightforward. In addition to being solitary hunters of small prey, cats are small prey themselves for other carni-vores, including dogs. Regardless of how sure the client is that others in the home will not hurt the cat, to the cat they may represent a threat. Providing the cat ways to escape at any time, including to vertical safe spaces out of reach of other pets and small children, often reduces its perception of threat to tolerable levels. For older children and adults, it usually suffices to explain that cats may not understand rough treatment as play, but as a predatory threat.

Chronic Pharmacotherapy

A variety of drugs have been recommended for use in cats with FIC, but to our knowl-edge no studies comparing their effectiveness with that of MEMO have been pub-lished. There also are hazards associated with drug therapy of cats, which include the aversion of many cats to chronic administration of oral medications, and potential unwanted side effects. With regard to drugs targeting anxiety in general, a recent re-view of behavioral psychopharmacology in cats[82] reminds us that, "There are no approved behavioral drugs for cats. Using any of the previously mentioned medica-tions for purposes other than the indications listed on the label and the use of any psy-choactive medication not listed previously is considered extra label use and falls under the rules of the Animal Medicinal Drug Use Clarification Act of 1994 and its implement-ing regulations." In fact, many drugs used for FIC are considered "off-label," and owner consent should be obtained before therapy. The review goes on to speculate that maropitant (Cerenia-Zoetis) "has the potential for many additional uses including as an adjunct medication for the treatment of pain and as a mediator of the stress response during handling and hospitalization." Unfortunately, there is no published ev-idence to support this speculation for cats, and currently available studies in other species suggest that effectiveness in the situations described is not highly likely.[83] There also is one (manufacturer-funded) 4-week study[84] of alpha S1 casein (Zylkene) in anxious cats, but the statistics reported leave one skeptical of the results, and no studies of cats with FIC have been conducted to our knowledge.

Although psychoactive drugs should not be used for cats on initial presentation for acute care of FIC,[85] they may be considered for cats if addressing their environmental needs does not resolve their clinical signs. We consider the use of tricyclic antidepres-sant and related drugs to be alternatives to euthanasia; to be used only when other approaches have failed. For example, amitriptyline (2.5–7.5 mg/cat PO every 24 hours) was evaluated in an open, non-placebo-controlled trial. It seemed to reduce clinical signs in some cats with severe, refractory FIC.[86] This drug, or clomipramine, another tricyclic antidepressant (0.25–0.5 mg/kg PO every 24 hours), may need to be admin-istered for weeks before a beneficial effect may be noted. If no improvements are noted, or medicating the cat is too stressful (for the owner or the cat), these drugs should be withdrawn gradually, over a period of 1 to 2 weeks. Side effects of the tri-cyclic antidepressants include sedation, lethargy, weight gain, and urine retention. Because of the possibility of urine retention, we advise monitoring the cat for stone development if clinical signs recur after receiving this class of drugs for an extended period. Fluoxetine (0.5–1 mg/kg PO every 24 hours) is a selective serotonin reuptake inhibitor. It has been shown to decrease signs of urine marking in cats.[87] This drug should also not be abruptly stopped. Selective serotonin reuptake inhibitor side ef-fects can include behavior changes, such as anxiety, and sleep disturbances.

Pentosan polysulfate sodium is a semisynthetic carbohydrate derivative similar to glycosaminoglycans that is also approved for humans with BPS/IC. A multicentered, placebo-controlled, masked study in cats found no significant differences when comparing pentosan polysulfate sodium with placebo.[88] However, all groups had clinical benefit, suggesting a strong placebo effect. All medication was provided to the cat in a food treat, leading some of the authors of the study to speculate that improving the interaction and environmental needs of the cat may inadvertently have contributed to the positive outcomes noted in all groups. Similar findings were reported in two other studies evaluating glycosaminoglycan therapy in cats with FIC,[89,90] and pentosan polysulfate has been shown to be equivalent to placebo in humans with BPS/IC.[91,92]

ADDITIONAL APPROACHES
Pheromones and Other Scents

Five facial pheromone fractions have been isolated from cats; cats deposit the "F3" fraction on prominent objects (including humans) by rubbing against the object when the cat feels safe and at ease.[93–95] Feliway, a synthetic analogue of this occurring feline facial pheromone, was developed to decrease anxiety-related behaviors of cats. Treatment with this pheromone (most often in company-funded studies) has been reported to reduce the amount of anxiety experienced by cats in unfamiliar circumstances, a response that may be helpful to these patients and their owners. Decreased spraying in multicat households, decreased marking, and a significant decrease in scratching behavior also has been reported subsequent to its use. In a pilot study evaluating Feliway in cats with FIC, no significant decrease in the number of days that clinical signs were exhibited was found.[96] Moreover, recent systematic reviews[97,98] and studies[99] have questioned its efficacy.

Another recent study reported that some cats may enjoy other scents, including catnip, silver vine, Tatarian honeysuckle, and valerian (a constituent of Feliway spray, but not diffusers). Another recent study reported that pet cat's preferences were: owner social interaction with the owner (50%) = food (37%) > toys (11%) > scent (2%). Preference for food was not different from toys, but greater than for scent.[100] Although social interaction with humans was the most-preferred stimulus category for most cats, followed by food, there was clear individual variability among the cats in preference, demonstrating once again the importance of "asking the cat" by offering changes as choices.

SUMMARY

Many indoor-housed cats seem to survive perfectly well by accommodating to less than perfect surroundings. The neuroendocrine-immune abnormalities in the cats with FIC, however, do not seem to permit the adaptive capacity of healthy cats, so these cats may be considered a separate population with greater sensitivity to their environments. Early intervention with MEMO could help prevent an initial episode, or to prevent a single episode from progressing to a chronic disease. Furthermore, gaining a better understanding of FIC (including the most accurate descriptive terminology) may help researchers, veterinarians, pet food companies, and clients develop and tailor the best possible approaches to management of these cat's unique health and welfare needs.

REFERENCES

1. Osborne CA, Johnston GR, Polzin DJ, et al. Redefinition of the feline urologic syndrome: feline lower urinary tract disease with heterogeneous causes. Vet Clin North Am Small Anim Pract 1984;14:409–38.

2. Kirk H. Retention of urine and urine deposits. The diseases of the cat and its general management. London: Balliere, Tindall and Cox; 1925. p. 261–7.
3. Osbaldiston GW, Taussig RA. Clinical report on 46 cases of feline urological syndrome. Vet Med Small Anim Clin 1970;65:461–8.
4. Barsanti JA, Finco DR, Shotts EB, et al. Feline urologic syndrome: further investigation into therapy. J Am Anim Hosp Assoc 1982;18:387–90.
5. Markwell PJ, Buffington CA, Chew DJ, et al. Clinical evaluation of commercially available urinary acidification diets in the management of idiopathic cystitis in cats. J Am Vet Med Assoc 1999;214:361–5.
6. Hanno PM, Erickson D, Moldwin R, et al. Diagnosis and treatment of interstitial cystitis/bladder pain syndrome: AUA guideline amendment. J Urol 2015;193:1545–53.
7. Clemens JQ, Meenan RT, O'Keeffe Rosetti MC, et al. Case-control study of medical comorbidities in women with interstitial cystitis. J Urol 2008;179:2222–5.
8. Parsons JK, Parsons CL. The historical origins of interstitial cystitis. J Urol 2004;171:20–2.
9. Buffington CA, Chew DJ, Woodworth BE. Interstitial cystitis in humans, and cats? Urology 1999;53:239.
10. Buffington CA. Idiopathic cystitis in domestic cats-beyond the lower urinary tract. J Vet Intern Med 2011;25:784–96.
11. Buffington CAT. Pandora syndrome in cats: diagnosis and treatment. Today's Veterinary Practice 2018;8:31–41.
12. Buffington CA. Developmental influences on medically unexplained symptoms. Psychother Psychosom 2009;78:139–44.
13. Warren JW, Howard FM, Cross RK, et al. Antecedent nonbladder syndromes in case-control study of interstitial cystitis/painful bladder syndrome. Urology 2009;73:52–7.
14. Nickel JC, Shoskes D, Irvine-Bird K. Clinical phenotyping of women with interstitial cystitis/painful bladder syndrome: a key to classification and potentially improved management. J Urol 2009;182:155–60.
15. Dinis S, de Oliveira JT, Pinto R, et al. From bladder to systemic syndrome: concept and treatment evolution of interstitial cystitis. J Womens Health 2015;7:735–44.
16. Birder LA, Hanna-Mitchell AT, Mayer E, et al. Cystitis, co-morbid disorders and associated epithelial dysfunction. Neurourol Urodyn 2011;30:668–72.
17. Buffington CA. Comorbidity of interstitial cystitis with other unexplained clinical conditions. J Urol 2004;172:1242–8.
18. Tai LW, Yeung SC, Cheung CW. Enriched environment and effects on neuropathic pain: experimental findings and mechanisms. Pain Pract 2018;18(8):1068–82.
19. Sant GR. Interstitial cystitis. Curr Opin Obstet Gynecol 1997;9:332–6.
20. Clasper M. A case of interstitial cystitis and Hunner's ulcer in a domestic short-haired cat. N Z Vet J 1990;38:158–60.
21. Lemberger SI, Dorsch R, Hauck SM, et al. Decrease of Trefoil factor 2 in cats with feline idiopathic cystitis. BJU Int 2011;107:670–7.
22. Parys M, Yuzbasiyan-Gurkan V, Kruger JM. Serum cytokine profiling in cats with acute idiopathic cystitis. J Vet Intern Med 2018;32:274–9.
23. Rubio-Diaz DE, Pozza ME, Dimitrakov J, et al. A candidate serum biomarker for bladder pain syndrome/interstitial cystitis. Analyst 2009;134:1133–7.
24. Parys M, Kruger JM, Yuzbasiyan-Gurkan V. Evaluation of immunomodulatory properties of feline mesenchymal stem cells. Stem Cells Dev 2017;26:776–85.

25. Birder LA, Barrick SR, Roppolo JR, et al. Feline interstitial cystitis results in mechanical hypersensitivity and altered ATP release from bladder urothelium. Am J Physiol Renal Physiol 2003;285:F423–9.

26. Sculptoreanu A, de Groat WC, Buffington CA, et al. Abnormal excitability in capsaicin-responsive DRG neurons from cats with feline interstitial cystitis. Exp Neurol 2005;193:437–43.

27. Birder LA, Nealen ML, Kiss S, et al. Beta-adrenoceptor agonists stimulate endothelial nitric oxide synthase in rat urinary bladder urothelial cells. J Neurosci 2002;22:8063–70.

28. Jezernik K, Romih R, Mannherz HG, et al. Immunohistochemical detection of apoptosis, proliferation and inducible nitric oxide synthase in rat urothelium damaged by cyclophosphamide treatment. Cell Biol Int 2003;27:863–9.

29. Kubes P. Nitric oxide modulates epithelial permeability in the feline small intestine. Am J Physiol 1992;262:G1138–42.

30. Cals-Grierson MM, Ormerod AD. Nitric oxide function in the skin. Nitric Oxide 2004;10:179–93.

31. Shim JS, Kang SG, Park JY, et al. Differences in urodynamic parameters between women with interstitial cystitis and/or bladder pain syndrome and severe overactive bladder. Urology 2016;94:64–9.

32. Wu CH, Buffington CA, Fraser MO, et al. Urodynamic evaluation of female cats with idiopathic cystitis. Am J Vet Res 2011;72:578–82.

33. Buffington CAT. External and internal influences on disease risk in cats. J Am Vet Med Assoc 2002;220:994–1002.

34. Westropp JL, Welk K, Buffington CA. Small adrenal glands in cats with feline interstitial cystitis. J Urologys 2003;170(6):2494–7.

35. Stella J, Croney C, Buffington T. Effects of stressors on the behavior and physiology of domestic cats. Appl Anim Behav Sci 2013;143:157–63.

36. Stella JL, Lord LK, Buffington CA. Sickness behaviors in response to unusual external events in healthy cats and cats with feline interstitial cystitis. J Am Vet Med Assoc 2011;238:67–73.

37. Westropp JL, Welk K, Buffington CA. Adrenal abnormalities in cats with feline interstitial cystitis. J Urol 2003;169:258.

38. Buffington CAT, Westropp JL, Chew DJ, et al. Clinical evaluation of multimodal environmental modification in the management of cats with lower urinary tract signs. J Feline Med Surg 2006;8:261–8.

39. Buffington CA, Westropp JL, Chew DJ. A case-control study of indoor-housed cats with lower urinary tract signs. J Am Vet Med Assoc 2006;228:722–5.

40. Freeman LM, Brown DJ, Smith FW, et al. Magnesium status and the effect of magnesium supplementation in feline hypertrophic cardiomyopathy. Can J Vet Res 1997;61:227–31.

41. Lund HS, Saevik BK, Finstad OW, et al. Risk factors for idiopathic cystitis in Norwegian cats: a matched case-control study. J feline Med Surg 2016;18:483–91.

42. Defauw PAM, Van de Maele I, Duchateau L, et al. Risk factors and clinical presentation of cats with feline idiopathic cystitis. J Feline Med Surg 2011;13:967–75.

43. Kim Y, Kim H, Pfeiffer D, et al. Epidemiological study of feline idiopathic cystitis in Seoul, South Korea. J Feline Med Surg 2018;20:913–21.

44. Cooper EJ. Feline lower urinary tract obstruction. In: Drobatz KJ, Hopper K, Rozanski E, et al, editors. Textbook of small animal emergency medicine. Hoboken, NJ: John Wiley & Sons; 2019. p. 634–40.

45. Segev G, Livne H, Ranen E, et al. Urethral obstruction in cats: predisposing factors, clinical, clinicopathological characteristics and prognosis. J Feline Med Surg 2011;13:101–8.

46. American Veterinary Medical Association. Animal welfare: responsibility & opportunity. American Veterinary Medical Association; 2018. Available at: https://www.avma.org/KB/Resources/Reference/AnimalWelfare/Pages/default.aspx. Accessed January 8, 2019.

47. Cutcliffe JR, Travale R, Green T. Trauma-informed care: progressive mental health care for the twenty-first century. In: European psychiatric/mental health nursing in the 21st century. Springer: Springer International Publishing; 2018. p. 103–22.

48. Stella J, Croney C, Buffington T. Environmental factors that affect the behavior and welfare of domestic cats (Felis silvestris catus) housed in cages. Appl Anim Behav Sci 2014;160:94–105.

49. Carney HC, Little S, Brownlee-Tomasso D, et al. AAFP and ISFM feline-friendly nursing care guidelines. J Feline Med Surg 2012;14:337–49.

50. Morgan KN, Tromborg CT. Sources of stress in captivity. Appl Anim Behav Sci 2007;102:262–302.

51. National Research Council. Thermoregulation in cats. In: Nutrient requirements of dogs and cats. Washington, DC: National Academies Press; 2006. p. 270–1.

52. Dorsch R, Zellner F, Schulz B, et al. Evaluation of meloxicam for the treatment of obstructive feline idiopathic cystitis. J Feline Med Surg 2016;18:925–33.

53. Tirlapur SA, Burch JV, Carberry CL, et al. on behalf of the Royal College of Obstetricians and Gynecologists. Management of bladder pain syndrome BJOG 2016;124:e46–372.

54. Herron ME, Buffington CA. Environmental enrichment for indoor cats: implementing enrichment. Compend Contin Educ Vet 2012;34:E1–5.

55. Frankel RM. Pets, vets, and frets: what relationship-centered care research has to offer veterinary medicine. J Vet Med Educ 2006;33:20–7.

56. Hannan AJ. Review: environmental enrichment and brain repair: harnessing the therapeutic effects of cognitive stimulation and physical activity to enhance experience-dependent plasticity. Neuropathol Appl Neurobiol 2014;40:13–25.

57. Vachon P, Millecamps M, Low L, et al. Alleviation of chronic neuropathic pain by environmental enrichment in mice well after the establishment of chronic pain. Behav Brain Funct 2013;9:22.

58. Hoy JM, Murray PJ, Tribe A. Thirty years later: enrichment practices for captive mammals. Zoo Biol 2010;29:303–16.

59. Heath S, Wilson C. Canine and feline enrichment in the home and kennel: a guide for practitioners. Vet Clin North Am Small Anim Pract 2014;44:427–49.

60. Lulich JP, Berent AC, Adams LG, et al. ACVIM small animal consensus recommendations on the treatment and prevention of uroliths in dogs and cats. J Vet Intern Med 2016;30:1564–74.

61. Bushnell MC, Case LK, Ceko M, et al. Effect of environment on the long-term consequences of chronic pain. Pain 2015;156:S42–9.

62. Reche AJ, Buffington CA. Increased tyrosine hydroxylase immunoreactivity in the locus coeruleus of cats with interstitial cystitis. J Urol 1998;159:1045.

63. Ellis SL, Rodan I, Carney HC, et al. AAFP and ISFM feline environmental needs guidelines. J Feline Med Surg 2013;15:219–30.

64. Carney HC, Sadek TP, Curtis TM, et al. AAFP and ISFM guidelines for diagnosing and solving house-soiling behavior in cats. J Feline Med Surg 2014; 16:579–98.

65. Newberry RC. Environmental enrichment- increasing the biological relevance of captive environments. Appl Anim Behav Sci 1995;44:229–43.

66. Laviola G, Rea M, Morley-Fletcher S, et al. Beneficial effects of enriched environment on adolescent rats from stressed pregnancies. Eur J Neurosci 2004;20: 1655–64.

67. Dandi E, Kalamari A, Touloumi O, et al. Beneficial effects of environmental enrichment on behavior, stress reactivity and synaptophysin/BDNF expression in hippocampus following early life stress. Int J Dev Neurosci 2018;67:19–32.

68. McMillan FD. Stress-induced and emotional eating in animals: a review of the experimental evidence and implications for companion animal obesity. Journal of Veterinary Behavior-Clinical Applications and Research 2013;8:376–85.

69. Kruger JM, Lulich JP, MacLeay J, et al. Comparison of foods with differing nutritional profiles for long-term management of acute nonobstructive idiopathic cystitis in cats. J Am Vet Med Assoc 2015;247:508–17.

70. Landsberg G, Milgram B, Mougeot I, et al. Therapeutic effects of an alpha-casozepine and L-tryptophan supplemented diet on fear and anxiety in the cat. J Feline Med Surg 2017;19(6):594–602.

71. Seawright A. A case of recurrent feline idiopathic cystitis: the control of clinical signs with behavior therapy. J Vet Behav Clin Appl Res 2008;3:32–8.

72. Turner DC. The human-cat relationship. In: Bateson DCTaP, editor. The domestic cat: the biology of its behaviour. 2nd edition. Cambridge (England): Cambridge University Press; 2000. p. 194–206.

73. Masserman JH. Experimental neuroses. Scientific Am 1950;182:38.

74. Dantas LM, Delgado MM, Johnson I, et al. Food puzzles for cats: feeding for physical and emotional wellbeing. J Feline Med Surg 2016;18:723–32.

75. Bateson P, Martin P. Play, playfulness, creativity and innovation. Cambridge, UK: Cambridge University Press; 2013.

76. McGowan RT, Ellis JJ, Bensky MK, et al. The ins and outs of the litter box: a detailed ethogram of cat elimination behavior in two contrasting environments. Applied Animal Behaviour Science 2017;194:67–78.

77. Horwitz DF. Behavioral and environmental factors associated with elimination behavior problems in cats: a retrospective study. Appl Anim Behav Sci 1997; 52:129–37.

78. Guy NC, Hopson M, Vanderstichel R. Litterbox size preference in domestic cats (Felis catus). J Vet Behav Clin Appl Res 2014;9:78–82.

79. Grigg EK, Pick L, Nibblett B. Litter box preference in domestic cats: covered versus uncovered. J Feline Med Surg 2012;15:280–4.

80. Herron ME, Buffington CAT. Environmental enrichment for indoor cats. Compend Contin Educ Vet 2010;32:E1–5. Available at: https://wwwncbinlmnihgov/pmc/articles/PMC3922041/.

81. Pachel CL. Intercat aggression: restoring harmony in the home: a guide for practitioners. Vet Clin North Am Small Anim Pract 2014;44:565–79.

82. Sinn L. Advances in behavioral psychopharmacology. Vet Clin North Am Small Anim Pract 2018;48:457–71.

83. Borsook D, Upadhyay J, Klimas M, et al. Decision-making using fMRI in clinical drug development: revisiting NK-1 receptor antagonists for pain. Drug Discov Today 2012;17:964–73.

84. Beata C, Beaumont-Graff E, Coll V, et al. Effect of alpha-casozepine (Zylkene) on anxiety in cats. Journal of Veterinary Behavior-Clinical Applications and Research 2007;2:40–6.

85. Kruger JM, Conway TS, Kaneene JB, et al. Randomized controlled trial of the efficacy of short-term amitriptyline administration for treatment of acute, nonobstructive, idiopathic lower urinary tract disease in cats. J Am Vet Med Assoc 2003;222:749–58.

86. Chew DJ, Buffington CA, Kendall MS, et al. Amitriptyline treatment for severe recurrent idiopathic cystitis in cats. J Am Vet Med Assoc 1998;213:1282–6.

87. Hart BL, Cliff KD, Tynes VV, et al. Control of urine marking by use of long-term treatment with fluoxetine or clomipramine in cats. J Am Vet Med Assoc 2005; 226:378–82.

88. Chew DJ, Bartges JW, Adams LG, et al. Randomized, placebo-controlled clinical trial of pentosan polysulfate sodium for treatment of feline interstitial (idiopathic) cystitis. J Vet Intern Med 2009;23:690.

89. Gunn-Moore DA, Shenoy CM. Oral glucosamine and the management of feline idiopathic cystitis. J Feline Med Surg 2004;6:219–25.

90. Wallius BM, Tidholm AE. Use of pentosan polysulphate in cats with idiopathic, non-obstructive lower urinary tract disease: a double-blind, randomised, placebo-controlled trial. J Feline Med Surg 2009;11(6):409–12.

91. Hanno PM, Wolf S. Guidelines Q&A: diagnosis and treatment of interstitial cystitis/bladder pain syndrome. In: Health policy brief. Linthicum (MD): American Urological Association; 2013.

92. Nickel JC, Herschorn S, Whitmore KE, et al. Pentosan polysulfate sodium for treatment of interstitial cystitis/bladder pain syndrome: insights from a randomized, double-blind, placebo-controlled study. J Urol 2015;193:857–62.

93. Pageat P, Gaultier E. Current research in canine and feline pheromones. Vet Clin North America Small Anim Pract 2003;33:187–211.

94. Bol S, Caspers J, Buckingham L, et al. Behavioral responsiveness of cats (Felidae) to silver vine (Actinidia polygama), Tatarian honeysuckle (Lonicera tatarica), valerian (Valeriana officinalis) and catnip (Nepeta cataria). BMC Vet Res 2017;13:1–15.

95. Pageat P, Gaultier E. Current research in canine and feline pheromones. The Veterinary clinics of North America Small animal practice 2003;33:187–211.

96. Gunn-Moore DA, Cameron ME. A pilot study using synthetic feline facial pheromone for the management of feline idiopathic cystitis. J Feline Med Surg 2004;6: 133–8.

97. Frank D, Beauchamp G, Palestrini C. Systematic review of the use of pheromones for treatment of undesirable behavior in cats and dogs. J Am Vet Med Assoc 2010;236:1308–16.

98. Mills DS, Redgate SE, Landsberg GM. A meta-analysis of studies of treatments for feline urine spraying. PLoS One 2011;6:e18448.

99. Chadwin RM, Bain MJ, Kass PH. Effect of a synthetic feline facial pheromone product on stress scores and incidence of upper respiratory tract infection in shelter cats. J Am Vet Med Assoc 2017;251:413–20.

100. Shreve KRV, Mehrkam LR, Udell MA. Social interaction, food, scent or toys? A formal assessment of domestic pet and shelter cat (Felis silvestris catus) preferences. Behav Processes 2017;141:322–8.

Urinary Tract Infection

Julie K. Byron, DVM, MS*

KEYWORDS

- Cystitis • Biofilm • Asymptomatic bacteriuria • Antibiotic

KEY POINTS

- Innate immune mechanisms are the primary defense of the lower urinary tract against symptomatic urinary tract infection.
- There are several options for in-house testing for urinary tract infection; however, many have been found to have drawbacks and must be carefully implemented.
- Asymptomatic bacteriuria is not an indication for treatment with antimicrobials and doing so may increase the risk of clinical infection as well as antibiotic resistance.
- Bacterial interference hold promise among several antimicrobial sparing treatments for urinary tract infection.

INTRODUCTION

Urinary tract infection (UTI) is a common diagnosis in companion animal practice. The incidence of UTI in the dog over its lifetime has been reported to be 14%[1] and in cats has been reported to be between 3% and 19%.[2–4] There are several factors thought to influence the risk of UTI in both species, including sex, age, comorbidities, and functional abnormalities of the lower urinary tract (LUT). There has been rising interest in characterizing the relationship of these risk factors to the development of UTI and bacteriuria. Point-of-care diagnostic testing for UTI has been evolving and improving therapeutic accuracy. A better understanding of the defense mechanisms of the LUT, the behavior of uropathogenic bacteria, and a growing awareness of the dangers of antimicrobial resistance have led to changes in the recommendations for diagnosis and treatment of UTI in dogs and cats.

Most of the UTIs in dogs and cats (~75%) involve a single agent, with *Escherichia coli* being responsible for up to half of the infections in dogs. This gram-negative organism is also the most common pathogen in cats (60%), with *Staphylococcus felis* being the most common Gram positive in that species.[5,6] A recent review from Italy found that gram-negative infections were more common than Gram positive and that there was more resistance to cephalosporins among these isolates than expected.[7]

Disclosure Statement: The author has received research support from Silver Lake Research Corporation, the manufacturers of RapidBact.
Veterinary Clinical Sciences, The Ohio State University, Columbus, OH 43210, USA
* 601 Vernon Tharp Street, Columbus, OH 43210.
E-mail address: byron.7@osu.edu

Vet Clin Small Anim 49 (2019) 211–221
https://doi.org/10.1016/j.cvsm.2018.11.005
0195-5616/19/© 2018 Elsevier Inc. All rights reserved.

vetsmall.theclinics.com

INNATE AND ADAPTIVE IMMUNITY OF THE BLADDER AND LOWER URINARY TRACT

The LUT has several mechanisms of defense against bacterial colonization. The innate immunity of the LUT is much better understood, and may be more important, than the adaptive immune functions. Prevention of ascending infection and mechanical removal of bacteria occurs in the ureters and bladder through the pulsatile flow of urine from the renal pelvis and the high shear flow of bladder voiding. In addition, there are several antimicrobial peptides that are expressed in the LUT, some in response to bacterial presence such as lipocalin-2, which prevents bacterial access to important mineral stores. The activation of the complement cascade and recruitment of neutrophils are also important parts of the LUT defenses. There is some evidence that if the host response is too vigorous and the development of inflammation too severe, there can be enough mucosal injury to take an acute UTI to a chronic state of inflammation and recurrent infections.[8,9] Immunocompromised mice that cannot mount a lymphocytic response in the LUT are also resistant to development of chronic cystitis. The addition of nonsteroidal antiinflammatory drugs (NSAIDs) in immunocompetent mice with recurrent UTI has shown to reduce this risk, even in animals with significant tissue injury.[10]

PATHOPHYSIOLOGY OF BACTERIAL CYSTITIS

The primary source of bacteria invading into the LUT is the colon and skin. The proximity of the rectum to the vulva makes this more common in female dogs and cats than in males. As in humans, the most common bacteria isolated from UTIs in the dog is E coli, followed by Staphylococcus species, Proteus, and Klebsiella. Enterococcus is often found as well, but most commonly as a secondary organism and will likely be cleared with treatment of the primary infection. Cats with UTI are primarily infected by E coli, followed by Enterococcus faecalis and S felis.

Bacteria in the LUT primarily exist in 2 forms, the planktonic state and the biofilm, which are phenotypically distinct and have differing host interactions and effects. Planktonic bacteria are free swimming in the urine and not adhered to any surface. They are generally more susceptible to many of the bladder defense mechanisms as well as antimicrobials but they also express different types of pili or fimbriae that facilitate adherence to inert and biological surfaces. Biofilms are structured communities of microorganisms within an adherent gel-like polymer, secreted by the organisms themselves.[11] They can form on the urothelium of the LUT or on inert surfaces such as urinary catheters and surgical implants. Biofilms are a frequent source of recurrent UTI in humans with indwelling catheters, and they present a challenge in dogs and cats with ureteral stents and subcutaneous ureteral bypass systems. The biofilm provides protection from antimicrobial substances through several mechanisms including decreased penetration, slow growth state of the bacteria, alterations in gene expression that confers resistance, and antibiotic binding/inactivation by polysaccharides in the matrix.[11,12]

Biofilms on inert surfaces begin with the formation of a "conditioning film" of components within the urine such as proteins and fibrinogen, which provide receptor sites for bacterial adhesins to attach. The bacteria sense the presence of an inert or biological surface through alterations in the concentration gradients of released signal molecules as they near it. A reversible adhesion of the bacteria occurs when the surface is encountered, which becomes irreversible with the formation of the biofilm structure. The biofilm is around 10% to 25% bacteria and 75% to 90% polysaccharide and water matrix with nutrient transport channels.[11]

The most widely studied bacterial biofilms in the urinary tract are those produced by uropathogenic E coli (UPEC). In the bladder, these bind to uroepithelial cells via uroplakins and $\alpha_3\beta_1$ integrins, which triggers neutrophil influx into the bladder lumen.

The host responds to interactions of the superficial epithelium with bacterial Type 1 fimbriae by triggering exfoliation of the epithelial cell with the attached bacterium and subsequent removal with the next urination. Some UPEC survive this defense mechanism by moving intracellularly and replicating to form intracellular bacterial communities. These can lay dormant or release back into the urine to resume a planktonic state and start the cycle over again. These IBCs survive by producing toxins and proteases that release nutrients from host cells and siderophores to retrieve sequestered iron stores as well as by inducing antimicrobial efflux pumps. The bacteria are safe from antimicrobial exposure but can trigger an innate immune response that involves expulsion of the organism by the host cell.[9] Some UPEC have the ability to establish deeper colonies in the bladder interstitium called quiescent intracellular reservoirs where they can stay dormant for months before reactivation. Some bacteria, such as *Proteus spp.*, will create a crystalline biofilm structure by producing urease and inducing struvite precipitation around the organism.[9]

RISK FACTORS

Whatever the organism, its ability to gain entrance to the LUT depends on an increased affinity for the environment of the bladder or a weakened host defense (**Box 1**). As noted earlier, female dogs and cats are at increased risk. One study in cats found females were 3.5 times more likely to develop an UTI than males. Several studies demonstrated an increased risk with increasing age and decreasing body condition score.[2,13,14] The inability to completely empty the bladder during micturition due to neurologic disease,[15] presence of urolithiasis, urinary incontinence, and immunosuppression have all been implicated as increasing risk of UTI in dogs and cats. Glucosuria has been shown to predispose dogs to emphysematous cystitis, a severe bladder infection with gas-producing organisms, but not to other types of UTIs.[16]

It has been a long held belief that decreased urine osmolality (ie, lower urine specific gravity) increased the risk for UTI due to dilution of substances that made urine a harsh environment for bacteria to grow. However, in recent years, this has been called into question because studies in cats have been unable to show a correlation with either clinical UTI or subclinical bacteriuria (SCB).[13] Dogs with a decreased urine specific gravity associated with hypercortisolism or diabetes mellitus did not seem to have an increased risk of UTI compared with those with more concentrated urine.[17] One recent in vitro study did note an increased ability to grow *E coli* in dilute urine,

---

Box 1
Identified risk factors for urinary tract infection and asymptomatic bacteriuria in dogs and cats

A list of some of the risk factors identified in dogs and cats for UTI and ASB.
  Female sex (D, C)
  Increased age (D, C)
  Decreased body condition score (D, C)
  Anatomic abnormality of the LUT (D, C)
  Functional abnormality of the LUT (D, C)
  Inability to empty the bladder (D, C)
  Urinary incontinence (D)
  Urolithiasis (D, C)
  Chronic kidney disease (D, C)
  Hyperthyroidism (C)
  Recent antibiotic use (D)
  Immunosuppression (D)

Abbreviations: C, cat; D, dog.

particularly if the urine was of acidic or neutral pH.[18] Further investigation is needed to determine the properties of urine that are most important as defenses against clinical UTI in the cat and dog.

The presence of a comorbidity may increase risk of UTI or SCB. In a recent study, among 194 cats with a positive urine culture, 78% had a comorbidity such as hyperthyroidism or chronic kidney disease (CKD). This study also found that cats with comorbidities were more likely to have SCB and those that were otherwise healthy were more likely to demonstrate clinical signs of infection.[4] The type of bacteria was also influenced by the presence of comorbidities. Healthy cats tended to have more *Staphylococcus* and *Streptococcus spp.* growth, whereas the cats with other systemic disease had more frequent *E coli* growth. There is some evidence that cats with CKD may have a higher incidence of SCB; however, this needs to be investigated further.[14] One study found that 17% of dogs with CKD had a positive urine culture, and of these, 45% were asymptomatic. It has been reported that in the healthy dog population, 2% to 9% of dogs have SCB, so it seems that CKD is associated with increased risk of SCB in dogs.[19] Whether this also indicates an increased risk for UTI has not been fully determined.

There is little information regarding the risk of UTI or SCB in dogs and cats that are treated with immunosuppressive drugs. Cyclosporine was shown to increase the incidence of SCB but not UTI in dogs treated for dermatologic disease with or without glucocorticoid therapy.[20] A similar study in cats found no association of glucocorticoid treatment, with or without cyclosporine, with either SCB or UTI.[21] It is not known whether the immunosuppression in the dogs prevented clinical signs of UTI by reducing the inflammatory response in the bladder or whether there were truly fewer uropathogenic colonizations. Anecdotal evidence suggests an increased risk of fungal cystitis, but the literature is limited to case reports.

SUBCLINICAL BACTERIURIA

There has been increased attention paid to what was once referred to as "occult UTI" but is now recognized as a subclinical bacteriuria. It has been recognized that the LUT is not a sterile site, and the urinary microbiome has begun to be defined in the dog;[22] however, most culture techniques of clinical urine samples are not sensitive enough to detect its components. Beyond the microbiome, there are a subset of dogs and cats that have a positive urine culture but do not have clinical signs of disease. In vitro and in vivo studies suggest that the host may have a genetic predisposition to a low response of the innate immune system to some of these bacterial strains.[23] Asymptomatic bacteriuria in humans is defined as the presence of bacteria with or without pyuria and lacking clinical signs associated with UTI, such as stranguria, pollakiuria, or suprapubicpain.[24] Standard of care is not to treat these patients with antimicrobial therapy unless they are pregnant or having invasive urinary procedures performed. There is strong evidence that the treatment of SCB does not decrease, and may increase, the risk of clinical UTI. It also promotes the development of antimicrobial resistance at a time when this is becoming a globally recognized problem.[25] Despite these guidelines, a recent study found that 17% of human hospital in-patient prescriptions of antimicrobials were for the treatment of SCB.[24]

The veterinary guidelines on treatment of UTI in cats and dogs indicate that SCB should not be treated.[26] The definition of SCB in dogs and cats has been under some debate. The potential for an owner to miss signs of discomfort and the subtlety of some clinical signs may lead to underdiagnosis of true UTI. In addition, there is a subset of patients, such as those with neurologic disease, which may not have enough sensory or motor function to display such clinical signs as stranguria or pollakiuria. It has been argued that the presence of pyuria should be considered a "clinical sign" in patients with otherwise asymptomatic bacteriuria and that these cases be treated as UTIs. On the other hand, there is currently no evidence that those dogs and cats with pyuria and bacteriuria that go untreated will develop worse outcomes, even in the presence of comorbidities such as diabetes mellitus or CKD.[2,4,27] A recent study indicated that treatment of UTI in dogs was the source of approximately 12% of oral antibiotic prescriptions in veterinary practice in the Netherlands.[28] With more attention to the recommendation to withhold treatment of SCB, and a better understanding of the drawbacks associated with unrestrained antibiotic use, the veterinary community has a chance to reduce the risk of antimicrobial resistance development.

CLINICAL SIGNS AND DIAGNOSTIC TESTING

A thorough history is important when assessing a dog or cat for UTI. The most common clinical signs associated with UTI are pollakiuria, stranguria, and hematuria. Fever is rarely found unless the animal has prostatitis or pyelonephritis. It is important to distinguish pollakiuria (small frequent urinations), in which the inflamed bladder will become painful with even small amounts of distension, and behavioral marking, in which the animal can hold urine and fill their bladder for an appropriate amount of time between urinations. Patients may exhibit discomfort on palpation of the bladder or around the kidneys or prostate if they have pyelonephritis or prostatitis associated with the UTI. Many dogs and cats will overgroom their genitalia or caudal abdomen when an UTI is present, potentially contributing to irritation of the penis or vulva that may be related to the underlying infection.

Diagnostic testing for UTI starts with a complete urinalysis, including specific gravity, urine chemistry, and wet-mount, unstained sediment examination under microscopy. The individual parts of the urinalysis have variable values in detecting an UTI in small animals. Urine specific gravity has not been shown to be a reliable indicator of an UTI in the cat[13] nor is it cost-effective to reflexively perform cultures on dilute dog urine if pyuria is not detected.[29] The urine dip strips used in evaluating urine chemistry are less accurate in detection of UTI in small animals than in humans. The nitrite test pads on some urine dip strips test for the presence of nitrate-converting Gram-negative bacteria in human urine. Unfortunately, the test is not reliable in companion animals. The leukocyte esterase test pad detects esterases in granulocytes; however, there is a high false-negative rate in dogs and a high false-positive rate in cats.[30]

The urine sediment evaluation is the most valuable portion of the urinalysis in detecting an UTI in the dog and cat. The combination of pyuria (>3–5 WBC/hpf) and bacteriuria on a urine sediment leads to a high index of suspicion for UTI. Unfortunately, the detection of bacteria on unstained wet-mount sediments is fraught with problems. The modified Sternheimer-Malbin urinary stain (Sedi-Stain, Becton Dickinson) is useful to highlight red and white blood cells and casts; however, it only stains dead bacteria, and bits of debris can be mistaken for organisms.[31] Several studies have found that examination of wet-mount preparations in both dogs and cats will overestimate the presence of bacteria in a urine sample. Gram staining and Wright-Giemsa staining of dry-mount preparations were found to have a higher specificity and positive predictive value in both dogs and cats.[32] In another study, the wet preparations of cat urine were found to have a sensitivity of 76% and specificity of 57%, whereas Wright-stained preparations had a sensitivity of 83% and a specificity of 99%.[31] In cats, it seems there are fewer false negatives than false positives using wet-mount, unstained preparations.[33] In dogs, wet-mount preparations were found to be inferior to Gram stain preparations, with a specificity of 66% versus 100%. Similar to the studies in cats, the wet-mount preparations had a 77% sensitivity, whereas the Gram-stained samples had a 96% sensitivity.[34] Although Wright-Giemsa and Gram staining of samples takes more time than preparing an unstained sample, it may reduce unnecessary culture and/or prescribing of antimicrobials in both dogs and cats.

The veterinary community has become more aware of the need for a reliable, rapid, and cost-effective point-of-care test for UTI in dogs and cats beyond the urinalysis. Several of these "bedside" diagnostics were developed for use in humans, and some have been investigated for use in dogs and cats. One test (AccutestUriscreen, Jant Pharmaceuticals), based on the presence of catalase in host cells as well as in many uropathogenic bacteria, was found to have an overall sensitivity of 89% and specificity of 71% in dogs and cats; however, it was still out-performed by the stained urine sediment examination.[35] A rapid immunoassay that differentiated between Gram-positive and Gram-negative bacteria in urine was evaluated in the dog and cat (RapidBac Vet, Silver Lake Research Corp).[36,37] It was found to have a 97% sensitivity and 99% specificity in dogs and a 79% sensitivity and 98% specificity in cats. The ability to determine gram-stain status of the bacteria is helpful to the clinician when choosing an appropriate antimicrobial without the benefit of a culture and antibiotic sensitivity profile. This diagnostic test may be useful in determining whether to perform a urine culture, especially in patients with sterile inflammatory urinary tract disease, such as cats with feline idiopathic cystitis.

Performance of in-house culture may also improve the ability of veterinarians to more accurately and cost-effectively diagnose and treat UTIs in dogs and cats. A urine culture paddle system (UriCult, LifeSign) was evaluated in dogs and cats and was noted to have a sensitivity and specificity of 89% to 97% and 99%, respectively for detection of bacteriuria; however, pathogen identification was only 76% accurate. It was also less accurate in samples with a low bacteria count. The investigators concluded the system may be of use but that the 24-hour wait time for test results was still not ideal.[38] Finally, a divided plate culture system (Flexicult Vet, Statens Serum), was evaluated on dog and cat urine samples.[39,40] Two studies found that it was highly sensitive and specific for detection of bacteriuria (sensitivity of 83% and specificity of 100%); however, the species identification accuracy was only 53% and highly depended on observer training. As with other culture systems, the delay in determining the presence of bacteria is less cost-effective if the test is unable to accurately identify the organism or determine its antimicrobial susceptibility. It is also important to remember that the accuracy of a test somewhat depends on the index of suspicion when performing it.

UNCOMPLICATED URINARY TRACT INFECTION

An UTI with clinical signs is generally considered "simple uncomplicated" or "complicated". Simple uncomplicated UTI is defined as occurring in an otherwise healthy patient with fewer than 3 episodes per year, no recent history of antimicrobial use, and a lack of underlying anatomic abnormalities of the LUT. Based on International Society for Companion Animal Infectious Disease (ISCAID) guidelines, the diagnosis of uncomplicated UTI includes the presence of clinical signs and a urinalysis with pyuria and bacteriuria. The guidelines recommend a quantitative urine culture be performed with suspected simple uncomplicated UTI.[26] Cultures should be performed on samples collected via cystocentesis or sterile catheterization. Free catch samples are only of value if the culture is negative. ISCAID guidelines recommend initial treatment of simple uncomplicated UTI be with amoxicillin or trimethoprim-sulfonamide for 7 days.[26] Little additional intervention is needed if clinical signs resolve during treatment.

COMPLICATED URINARY TRACT INFECTION

Complicated UTI involves an anatomic or functional problem with the LUT or a comorbidity that will increase the risk of UTI in a patient, including recent antibiotic use. Recurrent UTI is defined as 3 or more UTIs in a 12-month period and is generally classified as either relapse or reinfection. Relapse is infection with the same organism within 6 months of a treated UTI, either because there is continued exposure to that particular organism or because there is a nidus of infection that has not been cleared or addressed. Reinfection is the recurrence of an UTI with what is presumed to be a different organism and is likely due to host factors such as impaired immune defenses or increased risk of infection. These can be difficult to distinguish, especially if the same species of bacteria is always present. Evaluation of the susceptibility pattern can help, but there can be drift in the susceptibility over time depending on selection pressures on the bacteria.[26] Few practitioners perform the DNA analysis that will verify reinfection with the same strain of bacteria.

The ISCAID working group recommends a urine culture on all patients with a complicated UTI.[26] In addition, an evaluation of the underlying comorbidities or functional/anatomic abnormalities should also be undertaken to determine if they are correctable. Improved control of hyperadrenocorticism, correction of ectopic ureters, and medical management of urinary incontinence can all decrease the frequency of complicated UTI. If the underlying cause is not apparent, imaging and potentially cystoscopic evaluation may be needed to find the abnormality.

Treatment of a complicated UTI should be delayed until a culture and antibiotic susceptibility evaluation is completed, if possible. This will help avoid development of resistance. Symptomatic treatment with NSAIDs or other pain control may be needed to bridge this time and keep the patient comfortable. If an antibiotic must be started before the results are reported, it is advised to choose either amoxicillin or trimethoprim-sulfonamide, as for a simple uncomplicated UTI. Some classes of drugs are present in higher concentrations in the urine than in the plasma. When choosing from the antibiotics that the bacteria are susceptible to, these should be given greater consideration, because the concentrations that the bacteria are tested against are related to plasma levels of the drug, not the urine concentration, and there is a significant difference, particularly with penicillin and fluoroquinolones. This can be especially important in cases of resistant bacterial UTI, where an intermediate susceptibility to one of these drugs may mean susceptibility at the levels achieved in the urine. Generally, treatment of complicated UTI is for 4 weeks. There is little evidence of the use of antibiotics flushed into the bladder as a treatment for bacterial UTI; however, it may be part of treatment for fungal UTI.

Monitoring of treatment of complicated UTI is important and consists of a urine culture 7 days after starting antibiotic therapy and 1 week after completing it. Treatment failure indicates a need for additional diagnostic investigation, as long as client (and patient) compliance have been established. It is not appropriate to simply choose a more broad spectrum antibiotic without looking into why the bacteria failed to clear when it was susceptible in vitro.

PREVENTION

The most important part of preventing an UTI is to eliminate predisposing and complicating conditions. In some patients, this is not possible, and clinicians must consider options for preventing infection. These include prophylactic antibiotics, nonantimicrobial inhibitors of infection, and the introduction of competitive, nonpathogenic bacteria.

Prophylactic Antibiotic Therapy

Few studies have evaluated the effectiveness of continuous low dose or pulse antibiotic therapy for the prevention of UTI in dogs and cats. One study compared the use of a short-acting (cefazolin) and long-acting (cefovecin) cephalosporin perioperatively on dogs undergoing hemilaminectomy on the incidence of postoperative UTI. No difference was found between the 2 groups.[41] Current ISCAID guidelines do not recommend the use of low dose or pulse antibiotic prophylaxis in dogs and cats for prevention of UTI.[26]

Cranberry

Type A proanthocyanidins are a class of chemicals found in cranberry extract. They have been demonstrated in vitro to inhibit the *E coli* P fimbriae adherence to the uroepithelium.[42] This has been shown to be effective against *E coli* isolated from dogs and prevents attachment to canine uroepithelium; however, in vivo efficacy has been disappointing.[43] In a recent study evaluating the use of cranberry extract versus placebo in dogs with thoracolumbar disc herniation, no difference in the incidence of UTI was found; however, there was a suggestion that antiadhesion activity in the urine may have a protective effect.[43] Similar results have been found in people with recurrent UTI.

Mannose

E.coli that are pathogenic to the urinary tract (UPEC) express type 1 pili, which have a fimbriae H (FimH). This mediates the adherence of the bacterium to the uroepithelium via the oligomannosides of uroplakin1alectin. R-D mannosides block the adhesion of FimH in both the urothelium and the endometrium in animal models and is well tolerated. Although there are no randomized controlled trials in dogs or cats, such studies in people have had promising results.[42]

Probiotics

Women with UTI have a very different vaginal microbiome from those without one. In people, the use of probiotics to "normalize" the vaginal flora has proved successful in managing chronic and recurrent UTI. However, this approach does not seem to be as successful in dogs and cats. It may be due to the similarity of the vaginal microbiome in dogs with and without UTI. The maintenance of a healthy LUT and prevention of UTI in the dog is likely less dependent on the vaginal flora.[44] Probiotics have not been extensively evaluated in dogs or cats as a preventive measure for UTI; however, this evidence suggests they may be less useful than in people.

Bacterial Interference

Several strains of *E coli* isolated from chronic subclinical infections have been evaluated for protection against UPEC strains in animal models and in humans. There is evidence that in people, deliberately induced bacteriuria with these nonpathogenic strains may protect patients with incomplete bladder emptying from recurrent UTIs.[45] It is thought that these low-virulence nonpathogenic bacteria compete with and decrease the risk of colonization with more pathogenic organisms, although the mechanism is undetermined.[5] One study evaluated the effect of *E coli* 2 to 12 strain in 9 dogs with recurrent UTI. Four of these dogs achieved clinical cure of active infection and 3 of those had no recurrence of UTI. The biggest challenge in the use of this therapy is maintaining the bacteria in the bladder once it is healthy.[46,47] Further investigation of this novel therapy in dogs and cats with recurrent UTI is warranted.

SUMMARY

There are new paradigms in the way we define, diagnose, and treat UTI in dogs and cats. The need for antibiotic stewardship and the recognition of SNCB in our patients is driving much of this change. New findings about the host response to colonization and better understanding of the planktonic and biofilm states of bacteria have revealed potential new antibiotic–sparing options for the future.

REFERENCES

1. Ling GV. Therapeutic strategies involving antimicrobial treatment of the canine urinary tract. J Am Vet Med Assoc 1984;185(10):1162–4.
2. White JD, Stevenson M, Malik R, et al. Urinary tract infections in cats with chronic kidney disease. J Feline Med Surg 2013;15(6):459–65.
3. Vapalahti K, Virtala AM, Joensuu TA, et al. Health and behavioral survey of over 8000 finnish cats. Front Vet Sci 2016;3:70.
4. Dorsch R, von Vopelius-Feldt C, Wolf G, et al. Urinary tract infections in cats. Prevalence of comorbidities and bacterial species, and determination of antimicrobial susceptibility to commonly used antimicrobial agents. TierarztlPraxAusg K KleintiereHeimtiere 2016;44(4):227–36.
5. Olin SJ, Bartges JW. Urinary tract infections: treatment/comparative therapeutics. Vet Clin North Am SmallAnimPract 2015;45(4):721–46.
6. Lund HS, Skogtun G, Sorum H, et al. Antimicrobial susceptibility in bacterial isolates from Norwegian cats with lower urinary tract disease. J Feline Med Surg 2015;17(6):507–15.
7. Rampacci E, Bottinelli M, Stefanetti V, et al. Antimicrobial susceptibility survey on bacterial agents of canine and feline urinary tract infections: weight of the empirical treatment. J Glob Antimicrob Resist 2018;13:192–6.
8. O'Brien VP, Hannan TJ, Schaeffer AJ, et al. Are you experienced? Understanding bladder innate immunity in the context of recurrent urinary tract infection. CurrOpin Infect Dis 2015;28(1):97–105.
9. Flores-Mireles AL, Walker JN, Caparon M, et al. Urinary tract infections: epidemiology, mechanisms of infection and treatment options. Nat Rev Microbiol 2015; 13(5):269–84.
10. Hannan TJ, Totsika M, Mansfield KJ, et al. Host-pathogen checkpoints and population bottlenecks in persistent and intracellular uropathogenic Escherichia coli bladder infection. FEMSMicrobiol Rev 2012;36(3):616–48.
11. Tenke P, Koves B, Nagy K, et al. Update on biofilm infections in the urinary tract. World J Urol 2012;30(1):51–7.
12. Hall CW, Mah TF. Molecular mechanisms of biofilm-based antibiotic resistance and tolerance in pathogenic bacteria. FEMSMicrobiol Rev 2017;41(3):276–301.
13. Bailiff NL, Westropp JL, Nelson RW, et al. Evaluation of urine specific gravity and urine sediment as risk factors for urinary tract infections in cats. Vet ClinPathol 2008;37(3):317–22.
14. Puchot ML, Cook AK, Pohlit C. Subclinical bacteriuria in cats: prevalence, findings on contemporaneous urinalyses and clinical risk factors. J Feline Med Surg 2017;19(12):1238–44.

15. Olby NJ, MacKillop E, Cerda-Gonzalez S, et al. Prevalence of urinary tract infection in dogs after surgery for thoracolumbar intervertebral disc extrusion. J Vet Intern Med 2010;24(5):1106–11.

16. Merkel LK, Lulich J, Polzin D, et al. Clinicopathologic and microbiologic findings associated with emphysematous cystitis in 27 dogs. J Am AnimHosp Assoc 2017;53(6):313–20.

17. Forrester SD, Troy GC, Dalton MN, et al. Retrospective evaluation of urinary tract infection in 42 dogs with hyperadrenocorticism or diabetes mellitus or both. J Vet Intern Med 1999;13(6):557–60.

18. Thornton LA, Burchell RK, Burton SE, et al. The effect of urine concentration and pH on the growth of Escherichia coli in canine urine in vitro. J Vet Intern Med 2018;32(2):752–6.

19. Foster JD, Krishnan H, Cole S. Characterization of subclinical bacteriuria, bacterial cystitis, and pyelonephritis in dogs with chronic kidney disease. J Am Vet Med Assoc 2018;252(10):1257–62.

20. Peterson AL, Torres SM, Rendahl A, et al. Frequency of urinary tract infection in dogs with inflammatory skin disorders treated with ciclosporin alone or in combination with glucocorticoid therapy: a retrospective study. Vet Dermatol 2012; 23(3):201-e43.

21. Lockwood SL, Schick AE, Lewis TP, et al. Investigation of subclinical bacteriuria in cats with dermatological disease receiving long-term glucocorticoids and/or ciclosporin. Vet Dermatol 2018;29(1):25-e12.

22. Burton EN, Cohn LA, Reinero CN, et al. Characterization of the urinary microbiome in healthy dogs. PLoS One 2017;12(5):e0177783.

23. Gronberg-Hernandez J, Sunden F, Connolly J, et al. Genetic control of the variable innate immune response to asymptomatic bacteriuria. PLoS One 2011; 6(11):e28289.

24. Flokas ME, Andreatos N, Alevizakos M, et al. Inappropriate management of asymptomatic patients with positive urine cultures: a systematic review and meta-analysis. OpenForum Infect Dis 2017;4(4):ofx207.

25. Trautner BW. Asymptomatic bacteriuria: when the treatment is worse than the disease. Nat Rev Urol 2011;9(2):85–93.

26. Weese JS, Blondeau JM, Boothe D, et al. Antimicrobial use guidelines for treatment of urinary tract disease in dogs and cats: antimicrobial guidelines working group of the international society for companion animal infectious diseases. Vet Med Int 2011;2011:263768.

27. Wan SY, Hartmann FA, Jooss MK, et al. Prevalence and clinical outcome of subclinical bacteriuria in female dogs. J Am Vet Med Assoc 2014;245(1):106–12.

28. Sorensen TM, Bjornvad CR, Cordoba G, et al. Effects of diagnostic work-up on medical decision-making for canine urinary tract infection: an observational study in Danish small animal practices. J Vet Intern Med 2018;32(2):743–51.

29. Tivapasi MT, Hodges J, Byrne BA, et al. Diagnostic utility and cost-effectiveness of reflex bacterial culture for the detection of urinary tract infection in dogs with low urine specific gravity. Vet ClinPathol 2009;38(3):337–42.

30. Reine NJ, Langston CE. Urinalysis interpretation: how to squeeze out the maximum information from a small sample. Clin Tech SmallAnimPract 2005; 20(1):2–10.

31. Swenson CL, Boisvert AM, Gibbons-Burgener SN, et al. Evaluation of modified Wright-staining of dried urinary sediment as a method for accurate detection of bacteriuria in cats. Vet ClinPathol 2011;40(2):256–64.

32. O'Neil E, Horney B, Burton S, et al. Comparison of wet-mount, Wright-Giemsa and Gram-stained urine sediment for predicting bacteriuria in dogs and cats. Can Vet J 2013;54(11):1061–6.
33. Lund HS, Krontveit RI, Halvorsen I, et al. Evaluation of urinalyses from untreated adult cats with lower urinary tract disease and healthy control cats: predictive abilities and clinical relevance. J Feline Med Surg 2013;15(12):1086–97.
34. Way LI, Sullivan LA, Johnson V, et al. Comparison of routine urinalysis and urine Gram stain for detection of bacteriuria in dogs. J Vet EmergCritCare (San Antonio) 2013;23(1):23–8.
35. Kvitko-White HL, Cook AK, Nabity MB, et al. Evaluation of a catalase-based urine test for the detection of urinary tract infection in dogs and cats. J Vet Intern Med 2013;27(6):1379–84.
36. Jacob ME, Crowell MD, Fauls MB, et al. Diagnostic accuracy of a rapid immuno-assay for point of-care detection of urinary tract infection in dogs. Am J Vet Res 2016;77(2):162–6.
37. Daniels J, MN, Byron JK. Evaluation of a rapid immunoassay for point-of-care detection of bacteria in cat urine. ACVIM forum proceedings 2017. Available at: https://www.vin.com/members/cms/project/defaultadv1.aspx?id=8011996&pid= 18492&. Accessed August 30, 2018.
38. Ybarra WL, Sykes JE, Wang Y, et al. Performance of a veterinary urine dipstick paddle system for diagnosis and identification of urinary tract infections in dogs and cats. J Am Vet Med Assoc 2014;244(7):814–9.
39. Guardabassi L, Hedberg S, Jessen LR, et al. Optimization and evaluation of Flex-icult(R) Vet for detection, identification and antimicrobial susceptibility testing of bacterial uropathogens in small animal veterinary practice. Acta Vet Scand 2015;57:72.
40. Uhl A, Hartmann FA, Viviano KR. Clinical performance of a commercial point-of-care urine culture system for identification of bacteriuria in dogs. J Am Vet Med Assoc 2017;251(8):922–8.
41. Palamara JD, Bonczynski JJ, Berg JM, et al. Perioperative Cefovecin to reduce the incidence of urinary tract infection in dogs undergoing hemilaminectomy. J Am AnimHosp Assoc 2016;52(5):297–304.
42. Raditic DM. Complementary and integrative therapies for lower urinary tract dis-eases. Vet Clin North Am SmallAnimPract 2015;45(4):857–78.
43. Olby NJ, Vaden SL, Williams K, et al. Effect of cranberry extract on the frequency of Bacteriuria in dogs with acute thoracolumbar disk herniation: a randomized controlled clinical trial. J Vet Intern Med 2017;31(1):60–8.
44. Hutchins RG, Vaden SL, Jacob ME, et al. Vaginal microbiota of spayed dogs with or without recurrent urinary tract infections. J Vet Intern Med 2014;28(2):300–4.
45. Sunden F, Hakansson L, Ljunggren E, et al. Escherichia coli 83972 bacteriuria protects against recurrent lower urinary tract infections in patients with incom-plete bladder emptying. J Urol 2010;184(1):179–85.
46. Segev G, Sykes JE, Klumpp DJ, et al. Evaluation of the live biotherapeutic prod-uct, asymptomatic bacteriuria Escherichia coli 2-12, in healthy dogs and dogs with clinical recurrent UTI. J Vet Intern Med 2018;32(1):267–73.
47. Thompson MF, Schembri MA, Mills PC, et al. A modified three-dose protocol for colonization of the canine urinary tract with the asymptomatic bacteriuria Escher-ichia coli strain 83972. Vet Microbiol 2012;158(3–4):446–50.

Stem Cell Therapy

Jessica M. Quimby, DVM, PhD

KEYWORDS

- Mesenchymal stem cell • Mesenchymal stromal cell • Feline • Canine
- Chronic kidney disease • Acute kidney injury

KEY POINTS

- Based on rodent models of renal disease, mesenchymal stem cell therapy has great potential as a therapeutic modality in veterinary medicine.
- In the small number of studies that have been performed in cats and dogs, results have been varied and additional definitive evidence of efficacy is needed.
- Mesenchymal stem cell therapy should still be considered an experimental therapy for canine and feline chronic kidney disease and acute kidney injury.

INTRODUCTION

Stem cell therapy is an innovative new field of scientific investigation and clinical application that holds promise for the treatment of a variety of diseases in veterinary medicine. Recent years have brought increased interest in the potential for adult stem cells to help in the treatment of many diseases through their regenerative properties as well as their apparent ability to alter the environment in injured and diseased tissues. In particular, adult stem cells, called mesenchymal stem cells (MSCs), can migrate to affected areas and may be able to support the growth of other stem cells as well as moderate the response of the immune system. This type of therapy may therefore be useful in acute kidney injury (AKI) and chronic renal disease (CKD); however, additional investigation is necessary.

"Stem cell" is a generic term referring to any unspecialized cell that is capable of long-term self-renewal through cell division but that can be induced to differentiate into a specialized, functional cell. Stem cells are generally divided into 2 groups, embryonic stem cells and adult stem cells. Adult stem cells can be obtained from many differentiated tissues, including but not limited to bone marrow, bone, fat, and muscle. Obtaining adult stem cells also does not raise ethical concerns, and most commonly, stem cells are obtained from bone marrow or adipose sources. For most studies, the

Disclosure Statement: Dr J.M. Quimby is a consultant/key opinion leader for Kindred Bio, Aratana Therapeutics, Zoetis, Purina, Hill's, Royal Canin, VetCell, and Recellurate.
Department of Veterinary Clinical Sciences, The Ohio State University, 601 Vernon Tharp Road, Columbus, OH 43210, USA
E-mail address: Quimby.19@osu.edu

adult stem cell in question is actually a MSC or mesenchymal stromal cell. MSCs are multipotent but not pluripotent, which means they can differentiate into some, or "multiple," but not all tissue types.[1]

MESENCHYMAL STEM CELL SOURCES

MSCs can be isolated from virtually every tissue in the body. In cats, sources of MSCs that have been explored for expansion and clinical utility include bone marrow, adipose, and fetal membrane tissues discarded from pregnant ovariohysterectomy.[2–5] The tissue source with the highest MSC proliferation potential appears to vary from species to species.[6,7] In cats, adipose-derived MSCs (aMSCs) were found to be easier to collect and superior in proliferative potential than bone marrow–derived MSCs (bmMSCs) and are considered by most to be the preferred source for cats.[4] Although most earlier studies of MSC therapy in AKI and CKD rodent models use bmMSCs, more recent studies indicate similar efficacy with aMSCs.[8,9] Characterization and immunologic properties also appear to be similar between the sources,[10] with recent literature even suggesting an added advantage of using aMSC for immunomodulatory indications.[11]

Various types of MSC products have being investigated as a novel therapy for kidney disease, including aMSCs expanded in culture and stromal vascular fraction (SVF). SVF is the initial product of adipose tissue processing and is the type of cellular product produced from point-of-care processors and several private companies. Although isolation and expansion in culture allow the expanded aMSC product to have a purer population of MSCs, the SVF product contains multiple cell types. These cell types are thought to include MSCs as well as a mixture of B and T lymphocytes, endothelial cells, fibroblasts, macrophages, pericytes, and preadipocytes.[12] Currently, not enough information is known about SVF to determine if a cellular product with a mixed cellular type is a therapeutic advantage or disadvantage. Culture-expanded MSCs (both bmMSCs and aMSCs) are the type predominantly used in the rodent model literature; however, more recent rodent studies have started to explore the therapeutic potential of the SVF cellular product with promising results.[13,14]

Stem cells that are harvested from the patient with the intention of administering them back to that patient are termed autologous MSCs. Stem cells that are harvested from healthy donors for administration to the clinical patient are termed allogeneic MSCs. The relative efficacy of autologous versus allogeneic cells is an area of controversy. Although allogeneic MSCs are immune-privileged and are not expected to incite an immune response, according to some investigators they may not be as effective as autologous cells.[15] It is argued that autologous MSCs may survive longer in the body in comparison to allogeneic cells, which could reduce efficacy of the latter. Decreased efficacy of allogeneic MSCs in comparison to autologous MSCs has been observed in one acute renal failure rodent study.[15] However, allogeneic MSCs have been widely used in experimental stem cell transfer investigations, including clinical trials in humans, with positive results.[15,16] The advantages of using allogeneic MSCs include sparing the patient from undergoing the harvest procedure as well as the use of MSCs from young healthy donor animals. Recent studies in humans and rodents support the view that MSC obtained from young healthy individuals have greater proliferation potential and have greater therapeutic potential than those collected from elderly diseased individuals.[17–20] Poor therapeutic potential of MSC from elderly patients is of particular concern for application to kidney disease because it has been demonstrated that MSCs obtained from uremic rats have reduced proliferation in culture, premature senescence, and decreased capacity to induce angiogenesis.[21–23]

MESENCHYMAL STEM CELL CHARACTERIZATION

MSCs are plastic-adherent and assume a fibroblast-like morphology during culture. They proliferate easily in culture and can be cryopreserved without loss of phenotype or differentiation potential[24]; however, whether cryopreservation affects their immunomodulatory capabilities has not been fully investigated. Cell surface marker characterization via flow cytometry differentiates them from hematopoetic cells, but no truly unique MSC molecule has been identified.[25] For the most part, feline MSCs have been reported to be CD44 positive, CD 90 positive, CD 105 positive, CD 45 negative, HLA-DR negative, and these markers are similar in both bmMSCs and aMSCs.[2,4,22,25–27] In part, the lack of definitive markers probably reflects the diverse lineage of MSCs and the fact that each MSC population reflects to some degree the characteristics of tissues from which they were derived. Most importantly, stem cells from both adipose and bone marrow sources possess the ability to differentiate into cell types of multiple lineages, including adipocytes, chondrocytes, and osteocytes demonstrating their multipotent potential.[1,25]

MESENCHYMAL STEM CELL IMMUNOLOGIC PROPERTIES

MSCs clearly modulate immune responses, as demonstrated by both in vitro and in vivo studies.[28,29] For example, MSCs are poor antigen-presenting cells and do not express MHC class II or costimulatory molecules and only low levels of MHC class I molecules.[1] Thus, MSCs are very nonimmunogenic and can be transferred to fully allogeneic recipients and still mediate their immunologic effects.[15] Among their other immunologic properties, MSCs inhibit lymphocyte proliferation and cytokine production, suppress dendritic cell function and alter DC cytokine production, and decrease interferon-γ production by natural killer cells.[1] In vitro studies have demonstrated that MSCs can produce growth factors, cytokines, and anti-inflammatory mediators, all of which could help maintain or improve kidney function and suppress intrarenal inflammation.[16,30,31] The ability of MSCs to suppress inflammation appears to be mediated both by secreted factors and by direct contact with inflammatory cells.[16,31] These properties of MSCs could potentially be harnessed therapeutically.

CLINICAL APPLICATION TO KIDNEY DISEASE
Background

The potential of MSC therapy has been illustrated by literally dozens of studies assessing MSC therapy in rodent models of kidney disease, although most studies have focused on models of short-term protection from AKI.[14,30,32–34] Most of these studies provide evidence that systemic administration of bmMSCs or aMSCs (both culture-expanded and SVF products) can help preserve kidney function in the face of acute insults, such as ischemic injury, toxic insult, and obstruction, and can also help reduce tubular injury and fibrosis.[14,30,32–34] Thus, the available data indicate that systemically administered MSCs can help improve or stabilize kidney function in AKI by a variety of mechanisms.

Fewer studies have investigated the effects of MSC therapy in CKD rodent models.[26,27,35–40] Rodent models of CKD are most commonly created by performing a 5/6 nephrectomy, and a limitation of these models is that frequently MSC therapy is administered a relatively short time after nephrectomy (days to weeks). In most CKD rodent model studies that have been performed, administration of both bmMSCs and aMSCs has demonstrated significant renoprotective effects, including reduction of intrarenal inflammatory infiltrate, decreased fibrosis, and glomerulosclerosis.[26,27,35,39,40] Parameters of kidney function and clinical health, including weight, creatinine, blood urea nitrogen (BUN), proteinuria blood pressure, and hematocrit, have also been demonstrated to improve as a result of MSC therapy.[26,27,35,39,40] Several routes of administration, intraparenchymal, subcapsular, intravenous, have been explored, and all seem to be effective. Multiple repeated injections of MSCs appear to be even more effective than single injections.[26,35]

The mechanism of action for the effects seen in kidney disease studies is thought to be paracrine in nature, coming from both anti-inflammatory capabilities and protection of vascular integrity as mediated by vascular endothelial growth factor (VEGF).[26,35,36,38,40] Profibrotic molecules and cytokines and proinflammatory cytokines, specifically transforming growth factor-β, monocyte chemoattractant protein-1, and interleukin-6 (IL-6), are found to be decreased in MSC-treated rodents, particularly when multiple injections are administered.[26,35] Anti-inflammatory cytokines, such as IL-10 and vasculoprotective factor VEGF, have been shown to increase as a result of MSC therapy.[35,36,38,40] Although this body of literature demonstrates the immense potential of MSC therapy for kidney disease, it remains to be seen if results of rodent models are translational to veterinary or human patients.

Chronic Kidney Disease

A series of pilot studies assessing the safety and efficacy of administration of MSCs for treatment of cats with CKD has been conducted.[3,41,42] The first MSC study in cats with CKD was a pilot study assessing the safety and feasibility of autologous intrarenal MSC therapy.[41] Six cats (2 healthy, 4 with CKD) received a single unilateral intrarenal injection of autologous bmMSC or aMSCs via ultrasound guidance. Two International Renal Interest Society stage 3 CKD cats that received aMSCs experienced modest improvement in glomerular filtration rate (GFR) and a mild decrease in serum creatinine concentration. Intrarenal injection of MSCs did not induce immediate or longer-term adverse effects, but it was concluded that the number of sedations and interventions required to implement this approach made it unattractive for clinical application. In the course of conducting this study, it was also determined that expanding sufficient numbers of autologous MSCs in culture from elderly diseased patients was very difficult and time consuming. A more recent study in which one healthy cat received an intrarenal injection of amniotic-derived allogeneic MSCs documented hematuria and significant stress as a result of the procedure, and this study also determined the technique to not be clinically feasible.[43]

The feasibility of intravenous (IV) administration of allogeneic aMSCs to cats with CKD was also investigated.[3] Stable CKD cats with no concurrent illness were enrolled in a series of pilot studies and received an every-2-week IV infusion of allogeneic aMSCs collected and cryopreserved from healthy young specific pathogen free cats. Six cats in pilot 1 received 2×10^6 cryopreserved aMSCs per infusion; 5 cats in pilot 2 received 4×10^6 cryopreserved aMSCs per infusion, and 5 cats in pilot 3 received 4×10^6 aMSCs cultured from cryopreserved adipose. Cats in pilot 1 had few adverse effects from the aMSC infusions, and there was a statistically significant decrease in serum creatinine concentrations during the study period. However, the degree of decrease in serum creatinine concentrations was judged not to represent a clinically relevant improvement.

Notably, adverse effects of aMSC infusion were observed in most cats enrolled in the second pilot study that were treated with MSCs taken directly from cryopreservation. Vomiting occurred in 2 of 5 cats during infusion and increased respiratory rate, and effort was noted in 4 of 5 cats. In contrast, cats in pilot study 3 that received aMSCs cultured from cryopreserved adipose did not experience any adverse side effects. Serum creatinine concentrations, urinary cytokines, and GFR did not change significantly in cats in either of the latter studies. Based on the accumulated results of the 3 pilot studies, it appeared that use of higher doses of aMSCs taken directly from cryopreservation was the source of the treatment-related adverse effects. The most likely explanation for this reaction is an instant blood-mediated inflammatory reaction, which results in clumping of the cells as they contact the blood and potential subsequent micropulmonary thromboembolism.[44]

A randomized, placebo-controlled, blinded one-way crossover clinical study assessing the efficacy of allogeneic MSCs expanded from cryopreserved adipose with repeated administrations has also been performed.[42] Four cats were randomized to receive 2×10^6 aMSC/kg IV at 2, 4, and 6 weeks, and 3 cats were randomized to receive saline placebo. Although administration of aMSCs was not associated with adverse effects, significant improvement in kidney function (as determined by serum creatinine and GFR by nuclear scintigraphy) was not observed in the weeks following administration.

The IV administration of allogeneic MSCs derived from amniotic membrane has been assessed in 9 cats with CKD that received 2 injections of 2×10^6 MSCs 21 days apart.[43] One cat experienced vomiting during the first administration, but otherwise the MSCs were well tolerated. A statistically significant but mild decrease in serum creatinine was seen with stable body weight over the course of the study. Mild improvement in proteinuria and urine specific gravity was also seen. However, studies with a control group are necessary to determine if changes are attributable to MSC therapy or normal variation in values.

Acute Kidney Injury

Application of aMSCs for AKI in a feline ischemic kidney model has been investigated in a study where adult healthy research cats underwent unilateral ischemia for 60 minutes.[45] One hour after reperfusion, 4×10^6 of one of the following were administered via jugular catheter: aMSCs (5 cats), bmMSCs (5 cats), or fibroblasts (5 cats). Three historical control cats that had previously undergone the ischemia model were used for comparison. A mild reaction of transient hyperthermia was noted in most cats within the first day of administration. No significant difference in the percentage of cats that developed AKI and no difference in serum creatinine, urine specific gravity, proteinuria, GFR, or histopathology were noted as a result of MSC administration in this model.[45]

In a much more promising study, MSCs derived from umbilical cord blood (ucbMSC) have been investigated as a therapy in a canine model of AKI.[46] In this study, AKI was induced in 14 male beagle dogs with IV injection of gentamicin (15 mg/kg every 8 hours for 2 weeks before day 0) and cisplatin (70 mg/m^2 once on day 0). On days 6 and 23 after cisplatin, 1×10^6 green fluorescent–labeled ucbMSC in 30 μL phosphate-buffered saline (PBS) were injected into the renal parenchyma bilaterally using ultrasound guidance (3 dogs). A control group received 30 μL PBS bilaterally (8 dogs), and an additional control group received no intervention (3 dogs). Renal parameters including creatinine and BUN were assessed twice weekly during the study period. The survival rate was significantly different between the 2 groups that received injections ($P = .007$) with all dogs in the ucbMSC groups surviving to study end compared with only 1 of 8 dogs from the PBS-injected placebo group. Serum creatinine was significantly different between the groups when the highest creatinine after induction of AKI was compared with the last creatinine ($P = .01$). All dogs that were not already deceased were sacrificed at 7 weeks. The presence of fluorescent-labeled ucbMSC was confirmed in the renal cortex on necropsy. On histopathology, administration of ucbMSC subjectively improved scores for tubular necrosis, shedding of tubular cells and glomerular necrosis.

SUMMARY

Although MSCs potentially have great potential applicability to kidney disease, there are still many questions to be answered regarding the logistics of MSC therapy. The optimal route of administration, the ideal source of MSCs, and the impact of tissue donor status (attributes such as age, disease status, and sex) on MSC function remains to be determined. In addition, the degree to which and the mechanisms by which allogeneic versus autologous MSC products would undergo regulatory supervision have not been established. None of the studies conducted in cats with CKD have been able to replicate the efficacy of MSC treatment reported in rodent models of experimentally induced CKD or AKI.[26,27,35,36] One explanation for differing results of MSC therapy in cats with CKD is that the chronic nature of feline CKD makes these patients fundamentally different from rodents with experimentally induced disease. Although rodent studies illustrate the potential of MSC treatment of kidney disease, results of these models should be interpreted with caution. At this time, MSC therapy for CKD in cats should still be considered an experimental and unproven therapy. Few studies have been performed assessing MSC therapy for AKI in cats and dogs, and results have been mixed, although encouraging. For both disease processes, additional research is needed to determine the clinical applicability of this potential therapy.

REFERENCES

1. Reinders ME, Fibbe WE, Rabelink TJ. Multipotent mesenchymal stromal cell therapy in renal disease and kidney transplantation. Nephrol Dial Transplant 2010;25: 17–24.
2. Martin DR, Cox NR, Hathcock TL, et al. Isolation and characterization of multipotential mesenchymal stem cells from feline bone marrow. Exp Hematol 2002;30: 879–86.
3. Quimby JM, Webb TL, Habenicht LM, et al. Safety and efficacy of intravenous infusion of allogeneic cryopreserved mesenchymal stem cells for treatment of chronic kidney disease in cats: results of three sequential pilot studies. Stem Cell Res Ther 2013;4:48.
4. Webb TL, Quimby JM, Dow SW. In vitro comparison of feline bone marrow-derived and adipose tissue-derived mesenchymal stem cells. J Feline Med Surg 2012;14:165–8.
5. Iacono E, Cunto M, Zambelli D, et al. Could fetal fluid and membranes be an alternative source for mesenchymal stem cells (MSCs) in the feline species? A preliminary study. Vet Res Commun 2012;36:107–18.
6. Kisiel AH, McDuffee LA, Masaoud E, et al. Isolation, characterization, and in vitro proliferation of canine mesenchymal stem cells derived from bone marrow, adipose tissue, muscle, and periosteum. Am J Vet Res 2012;73:1305–17.
7. Ribitsch I, Burk J, Delling U, et al. Basic science and clinical application of stem cells in veterinary medicine. Adv Biochem Eng Biotechnol 2010;123:219–63.
8. Kim JH, Park DJ, Yun JC, et al. Human adipose tissue-derived mesenchymal stem cells protect kidneys from cisplatin nephrotoxicity in rats. Am J Physiol Renal Physiol 2012;302:F1141–50.

9. Furuichi K, Shintani H, Sakai Y, et al. Effects of adipose-derived mesenchymal cells on ischemia-reperfusion injury in kidney. Clin Exp Nephrol 2012;16:679–89.
10. Strioga M, Viswanathan S, Darinskas A, et al. Same or not the same? Comparison of adipose tissue-derived versus bone marrow-derived mesenchymal stem and stromal cells. Stem CellS Dev 2012;21:2724–52.
11. Ivanova-Todorova E, Bochev I, Mourdjeva M, et al. Adipose tissue-derived mesenchymal stem cells are more potent suppressors of dendritic cells differentiation compared to bone marrow-derived mesenchymal stem cells. Immunol Lett 2009;126:37–42.
12. Gimble JM, Bunnell BA, Guilak F. Human adipose-derived cells: an update on the transition to clinical translation. Regen Med 2012;7:225–35.
13. Riordan NH, Ichim TE, Min WP, et al. Non-expanded adipose stromal vascular fraction cell therapy for multiple sclerosis. J Transl Med 2009;7:29.
14. Yasuda K, Ozaki T, Saka Y, et al. Autologous cell therapy for cisplatin-induced acute kidney injury by using non-expanded adipose tissue-derived cells. Cytotherapy 2012;14:1089–100.
15. Togel F, Cohen A, Zhang P, et al. Autologous and allogeneic marrow stromal cells are safe and effective for the treatment of acute kidney injury. Stem Cells Dev 2009;18:475–85.
16. McTaggart SJ, Atkinson K. Mesenchymal stem cells: immunobiology and therapeutic potential in kidney disease. Nephrology (Carlton) 2007;12:44–52.
17. Scruggs BA, Semon JA, Zhang X, et al. Age of the donor reduces the ability of human adipose-derived stem cells to alleviate symptoms in the experimental autoimmune encephalomyelitis mouse model. Stem Cells Transl Med 2013;2: 797–807.
18. Lei L, Liao W, Sheng P, et al. Biological character of human adipose-derived adult stem cells and influence of donor age on cell replication in culture. Sci China C Life Sci 2007;50:320–8.
19. Kretlow JD, Jin YQ, Liu W, et al. Donor age and cell passage affects differentiation potential of murine bone marrow-derived stem cells. BMC Cell Biol 2008;9: 60.
20. Wang J, Liao L, Wang S, et al. Cell therapy with autologous mesenchymal stem cells-how the disease process impacts clinical considerations. Cytotherapy 2013;15:893–904.
21. Noh H, Yu MR, Kim HJ, et al. Uremia induces functional incompetence of bone marrow-derived stromal cells. Nephrol Dial Transplant 2012;27:218–25.
22. Klinkhammer BM, Kramann R, Mallau M, et al. Mesenchymal stem cells from rats with chronic kidney disease exhibit premature senescence and loss of regenerative potential. PLoS One 2014;9:e92115.
23. Idziak M, Pedzisz P, Burdzinska A, et al. Uremic toxins impair human bone marrow-derived mesenchymal stem cells functionality in vitro. Exp Toxicol Pathol 2014;66:187–94.
24. Martinello T, Bronzini I, Maccatrozzo L, et al. Canine adipose-derived-mesenchymal stem cells do not lose stem features after a long-term cryopreservation. Res Vet Sci 2011;91:18–24.
25. Schaffler A, Buchler C. Concise review: adipose tissue-derived stromal cells–basic and clinical implications for novel cell-based therapies. Stem Cells 2007; 25:818–27.
26. Semedo P, Correa-Costa M, Antonio Cenedeze M, et al. Mesenchymal stem cells attenuate renal fibrosis through immune modulation and remodeling properties in a rat remnant kidney model. Stem Cells 2009;27:3063–73.

27. Cavaglieri RC, Martini D, Sogayar MC, et al. Mesenchymal stem cells delivered at the subcapsule of the kidney ameliorate renal disease in the rat remnant kidney model. Transplant Proc 2009;41:947–51.

28. English K, Barry FP, Mahon BP. Murine mesenchymal stem cells suppress dendritic cell migration, maturation and antigen presentation. Immunol Lett 2008; 115:50–8.

29. McIntosh KR, Frazier T, Rowan BG, et al. Evolution and future prospects of adipose-derived immunomodulatory cell therapeutics. Expert Rev Clin Immunol 2013;9:175–84.

30. Togel F, Weiss K, Yang Y, et al. Vasculotropic, paracrine actions of infused mesenchymal stem cells are important to the recovery from acute kidney injury. Am J Physiol Renal Physiol 2007;292:F1626–35.

31. Barry FP, Murphy JM, English K, et al. Immunogenicity of adult mesenchymal stem cells: lessons from the fetal allograft. Stem Cells Dev 2005;14:252–65.

32. Semedo P, Wang PM, Andreucci TH, et al. Mesenchymal stem cells ameliorate tissue damages triggered by renal ischemia and reperfusion injury. Transplant Proc 2007;39:421–3.

33. Morigi M, Imberti B, Zoja C, et al. Mesenchymal stem cells are renotropic, helping to repair the kidney and improve function in acute renal failure. J Am Soc Nephrol 2004;15:1794–804.

34. Little MH, Rae FK. Review article: Potential cellular therapies for renal disease: can we translate results from animal studies to the human condition? Nephrology (Carlton) 2009;14:544–53.

35. Lee SR, Lee SH, Moon JY, et al. Repeated administration of bone marrow-derived mesenchymal stem cells improved the protective effects on a remnant kidney model. Ren Fail 2010;32:840–8.

36. Villanueva S, Ewertz E, Carrion F, et al. Mesenchymal stem cell injection ameliorates chronic renal failure in a rat model. Clin Sci 2011;121:489–99.

37. Kirpatovskii VI, Kazachenko AV, Plotnikov EY, et al. Functional aftereffects of intraparenchymatous injection of human fetal stem and progenitor cells to rats with chronic and acute renal failure. Bull Exp Biol Med 2006;141:500–6.

38. Choi S, Park M, Kim J, et al. The role of mesenchymal stem cells in the functional improvement of chronic renal failure. Stem Cells Dev 2009;18:521–9.

39. Ninichuk V, Gross O, Segerer S, et al. Multipotent mesenchymal stem cells reduce interstitial fibrosis but do not delay progression of chronic kidney disease in collagen4A3-deficient mice. Kidney Int 2006;70:121–9.

40. Villanueva S, Carreno JE, Salazar L, et al. Human mesenchymal stem cells derived from adipose tissue reduce functional and tissue damage in a rat model of chronic renal failure. Clin Sci 2013;125:199–210.

41. Quimby JM, Webb TL, Gibbons DS, et al. Evaluation of intrarenal mesenchymal stem cell injection for treatment of chronic kidney disease in cats: a pilot study. J Feline Med Surg 2011;13:418–26.

42. Quimby JM, Webb TL, Randall E, et al. Assessment of intravenous adipose-derived allogeneic mesenchymal stem cells for the treatment of feline chronic kidney disease: a randomized, placebo-controlled clinical trial in eight cats. J Feline Med Surg 2016;18:165–71.

43. Vidane AS, Pinheiro AO, Casals JB, et al. Transplantation of amniotic membrane-derived multipotent cells ameliorates and delays the progression of chronic kidney disease in cats. Reprod Domest Anim 2017;52(Suppl 2):316–26.

44. Moll G, Rasmusson-Duprez I, von Bahr L, et al. Are therapeutic human mesenchymal stromal cells compatible with human blood? Stem Cells 2012;30:1565–74.
45. Rosselli DD, Mumaw JL, Dickerson V, et al. Efficacy of allogeneic mesenchymal stem cell administration in a model of acute ischemic kidney injury in cats. Res Vet Sci 2016;108:18–24.
46. Lee SJ, Ryu MO, Seo MS, et al. Mesenchymal Stem cells contribute to improvement of renal function in a canine kidney injury model. In Vivo 2017;31:1115–24.

Importance of Urinalysis

Tara L. Piech, DVM, MS*, Kathryn L. Wycislo, DVM, PhD

KEYWORDS

- Urinalysis • Specific gravity • Urine chemistry • Proteinuria • Bacteriuria • Casts
- Crystals

KEY POINTS

- In addition to the identification of urinary tract disorders, a urinalysis is an indispensable test that can also aid in the diagnosis of nonurinary tract disorders, and it should be performed in both healthy and ill patients.
- Many renal and nonrenal factors can influence a patient's urine specific gravity. Therefore, urine specific gravity should be interpreted in light of hydration status, electrolyte concentrations, urea nitrogen and creatinine concentrations, and possible medications or fluid therapy.
- Not all results from a dipstrip or sediment examination are significant in every patient. As an example, low numbers of casts observed in the urine of an otherwise healthy patient may not be clinically relevant.

INTRODUCTION

Although overlooked by some practitioners, a complete urinalysis is often considered to be the single most important diagnostic test by many veterinary specialists. In addition to the identification of urinary tract disorders, such as bacterial cystitis, protein-losing nephropathy, and transitional cell carcinoma, a urinalysis can aid in the diagnosis of nonurinary tract disorders. Endocrinopathies such as diabetes mellitus and other systemic disorders such as intravascular hemolysis can often be diagnosed through urine evaluation.

A complete urinalysis consists of the assessment of color and clarity, measurement of urine specific gravity (USG), chemical analysis of urine, and microscopic examination of a urine sediment. It is important to remember that the results of these tests should be interpreted together rather than in isolation, considering pertinent patient clinical history and other physical examination findings. Urine should be at room temperature before evaluation to ensure accurate results[1] and should be analyzed within

The authors have no conflicts of interest to disclose.
Department of Pathology and Population Medicine, Midwestern University College of Veterinary Medicine, 5715 West Utopia Road, Glendale, AZ 85308, USA
* Corresponding author.
E-mail address: tpiech@midwestern.edu

Vet Clin Small Anim 49 (2019) 233–245
https://doi.org/10.1016/j.cvsm.2018.10.005
0195-5616/19/© 2018 Elsevier Inc. All rights reserved.

vetsmall.theclinics.com

60 minutes of collection to avoid temperature- and time-dependent effects on crystal formation.[2]

COLOR AND CLARITY

Urine from healthy dogs and cats normally ranges in color from light yellow to amber. Color can be influenced by diet, medications, and hydration status. For instance, a dehydrated patient may void a small amount of dark yellow urine in comparison with a euhydrated animal. A variety of pigments may also be present in urine, but pigmenturia related to the presence of hemoglobin, myoglobin, or bilirubin are most common and can impart a red to orange hue. It is important to note that these pigments are likely to interfere with certain urinalysis results, particularly of the dipstrip examination. Suspicion of hematuria should always be confirmed with a sediment examination to assess for the presence of erythrocytes.[3]

Urine clarity is typically graded on a subjective scale from clear to flocculent, and generally correlates with the amount of particulate material present in the sample. For instance, a high concentration of leukocytes, crystals, amorphous material, and/or microorganisms often lead to increased urine turbidity. The specific cause(s) of the turbidity should be determined by microscope examination of urine sediment.[3]

URINE SPECIFIC GRAVITY

USG is used clinically to provide an estimate of the ability of the renal tubules to concentrate or dilute the glomerular filtrate. It represents the ratio of a solution's weight to the weight of an equal volume of water.[4] Clinically, standard refractometers are commonly used to measure the refractive index of urine and provide an estimation of a patient's USG.[4] Many refractometers report USG results over a range of 1.000 (the USG of pure water) to approximately 1.040. If a patient's USG reads greater than 1.040, commercial laboratories will typically dilute the sample with an equal volume of pure water to obtain a result within the scale range, and then use the employed dilution factor to calculate the USG. To avoid having to perform this dilution step, Tvedten and Noren[5] investigated the usefulness and accuracy of a digital refractometer over a manual handheld Goldberg-type refractometer. The digital refractometer reported USG over a wider range of 1.000 to 1.080.[5] It was discovered that, compared with the Goldberg-type refractometer, the digital refractometer consistently underestimated USG.[5] This finding has important clinical implications, because it could potentially lead to a misdiagnosis of kidney or endocrine disease. Many refractometers are calibrated for specific species. If a human or canine-calibrated refractometer is used to measure the USG of feline urine, the USG may be mildly overestimated.[4] USG is typically not altered by sample storage time or temperature.[2]

USG is also a component of most urine reagent dipstrip systems; however, use of these strips to estimate USG is considered unreliable and not recommended in domestic animals.[4] Published normal reference intervals for USG include 1.015 to 1.045 for canines and 1.035 to 1.060 for felines.[3] However, a patient's USG should be interpreted clinically in light of hydration status, electrolyte concentrations, and urea nitrogen and creatinine concentrations, as well as possible medication (such as diuretic) or fluid therapy administration.[3]

Isosthenuria is defined as a USG between approximately 1.008 and 1.013 and indicates that urine osmolality is equal to that of plasma. The presence of isosthenuria in conjunction with an azotemia is strongly indicative of kidney disease. Hyposthenuria is defined as a USG of less than 1.007 and indicates a lack urine of concentrating ability that is not due to kidney dysfunction. Examples of disorders associated with hyposthenuria include central or nephrogenic diabetes insipidus.[4] It is important to note that marked glucosuria, such as in patients with hyperosmolar hyperglycemia (serum osmolality of >310 mOsm/kg)[6] or marked proteinuria may have a falsely increased USG. It is reported that USG can increase by approximately 0.005 for every 1 g/dL of glucose or protein in urine.[7]

CHEMICAL ANALYSIS OF URINE

Chemical analysis of urine is most commonly performed semiquantitatively by use of reagent dipstrip systems. The results of individual reagent pads on dipstrips are typically graded on scales (usually negative to 3+ or 4+) provided by the manufacturer. These strips can either be visually interpreted or analyzed by automated methods, which most commonly implement reflectance photometry.[4] Several recent studies reported good agreement between visual estimation and automatic measurements for most parameters.[8,9] In general, urine dipstrips are reliable for the measurement of urine pH, glucose, ketones, bilirubin, occult blood, and protein. They are considered unreliable for measurement of USG and leukocytes,[10] which should be assessed by refractometry and a microscopic sediment examination, respectively. Nitrite and urobilinogen measurements are also not typically reported in veterinary medicine.

pH

Urine pH is generally used to provide an overall estimate of a patient's acid–base status.[11] In addition to reagent pad systems, urine pH may be measured by a pH meter. A recent study found good overall agreement between urine pH measurement by pH meters and urine dipstrip methods in sheep, whereas a pH meter is more accurate in canines.[12] Urine pH is influenced by many renal and extrarenal factors, including diet, bacterial infection, and systemic illness. Canines and felines typically consume high-protein diets and therefore have more acidic urine (reference interval, 6.0–7.5).[4] However, both species may have alkaline urine postprandially owing to buffering in response to gastric acid secretion.[11] Urine pH can alter the results of a urine sediment; for instance, alkaline urine can result in struvite crystalluria as well as erythrocyte and leukocyte degradation.[3] Urine pH is typically not altered by sample storage time and temperature.[2] However, urine pH may have an effect on the in vitro growth of *Escherichia coli* organisms; 1 study reported that neutral to acidic, dilute urine results in higher log colony-forming units per milliliter than does alkaline, concentrated urine.[13]

Aciduria indicates increased kidney secretion of hydrogen ions.[4] Potential causes for aciduria include metabolic acidosis disorders, furosemide therapy, and proximal renal tubular acidosis.[4] Conversely, alkalinuria indicates decreased kidney excretion of hydrogen ions.[4] This may occur owing to spontaneous urea degradation from delayed processing of a urine sample. This also commonly occurs owing to the presence of urease-containing bacterial infections (such as *Staphylococcus* spp.), which form ammonium ions.[4]

Glucose

Glucose is present in the glomerular filtrate and in health is 100% reabsorbed by the proximal tubule; therefore, glucose is normally not present in urine at levels detected by reagent dipstrips.[14] A small degree of glucosuria may be present postprandially or owing to excitement or stress in felines.[11] When a patient's blood glucose concentration exceeds the renal threshold, glucosuria will occur.[14] Reported renal glucose thresholds are 180 to 220 mg/dL for canines and 200 to 280 mg/dL for felines.[14] Hyperglycemia with concurrent glucosuria occurs in disorders such as diabetes mellitus, hyperadrenocorticism, and acromegaly, as well as stress and therapy with dextrose-containing fluids.[14] Glucosuria with normoglycemia may indicate proximal tubular damage as can occur in conditions, such as Fanconi syndrome, hypoxia, drugs such as aminoglycosides, or toxins such as ethylene glycol.[14] On urine reagent dipstrips, false-positive glucose readings can occur owing to contamination with hypochlorite and hydrogen peroxide. False-negative readings can result from the presence of ascorbic acid or tetracycline therapy.[14] A relatively new product for felines, Purina Glucotest, is an enzymatic test that estimates glucose concentration in feline urine over 8 hours and is marketed as a litter additive designed to avoid feline urine collection. One study showed good agreement between the Glucotest and urine dipstrip methods at detecting glucosuria when the Glucotest was interpreted between 30 minutes and 8 hours after urine exposure.[15]

Ketones

Ketonuria is typically present when the body is in a state of negative energy balance and metabolizes fats rather than glucose. Ketonuria occurs in diabetic ketoacidosis, prolonged fasting or starvation, and consumption of low carbohydrate diets.[1] Most urine dipstrips detect both acetone and acetoacetate and are more sensitive to acetoacetate, but do not detect beta-hydroxybutyrate.[14] False-positive reactions may occur in highly pigmented urine, in the presence of levodopa metabolites, or in urine with a high USG and low pH.[4] Prolonged ketonuria may lead to hyponatremia and hypokalemia owing to kidney excretion of these electrolytes.[4]

Bilirubin

Bilirubin measured by the urine dipstrips represents conjugated bilirubin,[11] and bilirubinuria often precedes hyperbilirubinemia in most species.[4] Trace to small amounts of bilirubinuria may be present in healthy dogs with adequately concentrated urine owing to their low kidney threshold for bilirubin, as well as the capability of their renal tubular epithelial cells to convert heme to unconjugated bilirubin, which is then excreted in urine.[4] Bilirubinuria in felines, even if present in only trace amounts, is usually indicative of an underlying disorder. Possible disorders in felines include hepatobiliary disease or intravascular hemolysis.[11] Bilirubin rapidly degrades in the presence of ultraviolet light and high concentrations of ascorbic acid; therefore, false-negative reactions may occur in aged or slowly processed samples under improper storage conditions.[11]

Occult Blood

A positive reaction for blood on urine dipstrips can indicate the presence of either hematuria (presence of intact erythrocytes within urine), hemoglobinuria (owing to lysed erythrocytes), or myoglobinuria from skeletal muscle damage.[16] These causes can be distinguished by macroscopic examination of the patient's urine, microscopic examination of the patient's urine sediment, and assessment of the patient's complete blood count and serum biochemical parameters. If intact erythrocytes are present, the blood reagent pad will appear sparsely to densely stippled positive, and erythrocytes will be present on microscopic sediment examination.[16] If hemoglobinuria is present, the urine will be pink to red in color and will not clear with centrifugation; however, the blood reagent pad will be diffusely positive, and the patient's plasma may be pink in color.

Both hematuria and hemoglobinuria indicate active bleeding within the urinary tract.[16] Hematuria and hemoglobinuria may also be present owing to intravascular hemolysis or may be a result of iatrogenic blood contamination when urine is collected by cystocentesis or catheterization. Myoglobinuria indicates active skeletal muscle damage or necrosis, and typically imparts a red to brown-tinged color to urine. Plasma should be discolored, and the blood reagent pad will be diffusely positive, similar to what is observed in hemoglobinuria. Myoglobinuria can be supported by an elevated creatine kinase and/or aspartate aminotransferase activity on a patient's biochemical profile.[16] False-positive blood results can occur in the presence of hypochlorite or pigmented urine (eg, bilirubinuria); false-negative results can occur in the presence of formalin or ascorbic acid.[16] Because false-negative results for both blood and glucose on reagent dipstrips can occur in the presence of ascorbic acid, some dipstrips also include semiquantitative estimates of ascorbic acid concentration.[17] The influence of ascorbic acid on urinalysis parameters is likely more relevant in human medicine owing to possible vitamin C supplementation[17]; to the authors' knowledge, these effects have not been well-characterized in veterinary species.

Protein

Normal urine contains little to no detectable protein owing to effective reabsorption by proximal renal tubular epithelial cells[16]; however, the resorptive capacity of these cells can become saturated or defective, leading to proteinuria.[16] Reagent dipstrips are most sensitive for the detection of albuminuria at concentrations of greater than 30 mg/dL.[16] Other proteins in urine, such as globulin and Bence-Jones proteins, may or may not be detected by this method.[16] Causes of proteinuria are generally classified into prerenal, renal, and postrenal categories. Prerenal proteinuria can result from hemoglobin owing to intravascular hemolysis, myoglobin owing to muscle injury, or acute phase proteins released owing to inflammation, fever, strenuous exercise, or Bence-Jones proteins (neoplastic or infectious disorders).[16] Renal proteinuria may be caused by glomerular disease, tubular disease, or possibly both. Postrenal proteinuria refers to protein entering the urinary tract distal to the renal pelvis; causes include infection, blood from trauma or neoplasia, or blood from the genital tract.[16] False-positive reactions can occur in highly buffered alkaline urine (pH > 8.0) or highly pigmented urine, whereas false-negative reactions can occur in the presence of nonalbumin proteins, or in acidic urine.[16]

Blood contamination within a urine sample may also contribute to proteinuria. However, several studies on urinary blood contamination in dogs found that significant proteinuria (2+ or greater) on the urinary dipstrip pad often does not occur until the urine sample is visibly pink.[18,19] Interestingly, yellow urine that contains blood (but is not visibly pink in color) may still have a significantly elevated urine protein to creatinine ratio compared with yellow urine without blood contamination, which may or may not result in a clinically relevant increase in urine protein to creatinine ratio.[19] If proteinuria is identified via dipstrip methods in a patient with an inactive sediment, it is recommended to repeat a full urinalysis and, if proteinuria is still present, to perform more quantitative tests such as a urine protein to creatinine ratio.

URINE SEDIMENT EVALUATION

Although a large amount of information can be obtained through the gross and chemical evaluation of a urine sample and measurement of USG only, a urinalysis is not considered complete unless a urine sediment examination has been performed. Urine sediment evaluation can provide the clinician with evidence of inflammation, infection, or hemorrhage within the urinary tract through the visual identification of leukocytes, bacteria, or erythrocytes. It can also alert to the presence of renal tubular disease, hereditary metabolic disorders, or specific disease processes, such as ethylene glycol toxicity or possible urolithiasis, when specific casts or crystals are observed. In some cases, urine sediment evaluation may also provide information regarding potential urinary tract neoplasia, such as transitional cell carcinoma or lymphoma. Some clinicians also monitor crystalluria in patients with a history of urolithiasis and may use sediment findings to help guide therapeutic decisions. In this section, common and unique urine sediment findings, such as cellular elements (leukocytes and erythrocytes), crystals, casts, and infectious agents are reviewed.

Urine sediments are prepared by centrifuging the urine sample at a low speed for several minutes to pellet the nonsoluble materials within the urine. After decanting off the majority of the urine supernatant, a drop of the resuspended sediment can be viewed as a wet mount using low magnification microscope dry objectives ($\times$10 and $\times$40–$\times$50). At least 5 to 10 fields of the wet mount should be evaluated at each magnification.[20] In commercial veterinary laboratories, urine sediment evaluations are typically performed on unstained sediment preparations. Some clinics (often private clinics) may choose to use a sediment stain, such as Sedi-Stain, to facilitate the identification and differentiation of particulate elements. However, sediment stains can introduce significant artifacts, which can sometimes be confused for bacteria. If sediment stains are used in practice, those reviewing sediments must have confidence in their ability to recognize and differentiate artifacts to avoid unnecessary additional diagnostic tests or therapies. Automated urine sediment analyzers have also been developed for veterinary use, such as the SediVue Dx, which may be practical in large hospital settings that process large numbers of samples.

Similar to chemical analysis of urine, sediment evaluation is semiquantitative, and results are often reported out using ranges (eg, 10–20 erythrocytes per high-power field) or subjective descriptors (eg, rare struvite crystals). However, practices that perform in-house urinalyses can increase the meaning of their urine sediment results by implementing a standard operating protocol for the preparation, evaluation, and quantification of urine sediments, to keep interpersonal variations to a minimum when performing sediment evaluations.

MICROSCOPIC ELEMENTS
Erythrocytes

Identification of erythrocytes on urine sediment examination (hematuria) should be correlated with dipstrip pad findings for occult blood. The urine collection method should also be considered, because cystocentesis or genital tract contamination of free catch samples may be important sources of blood contamination. Erythrocytes will appear smooth and may be round, biconcave, or crenated and are typically approximately one-half of the size of leukocytes (**Fig. 1**). They may be colorless to slightly colored. In general, fewer than 5 erythrocytes per high-power field is considered to be a normal finding.[21]

Leukocytes

The presence of increased numbers of leukocytes in the urine sediment (pyuria) can be an indicator of inflammation and potential infection within the urinary tract, such as cystitis or pyelonephritis. On sediment examination, leukocytes are typically twice the size of erythrocytes and often have a granular appearance (**Fig. 2**). Similar to erythrocytes, fewer than 5 leukocytes per high powered field is considered a normal finding.[21] However, leukocyte numbers in urine may be elevated beyond this level in cases with significant hemorrhage or blood contamination and may not represent true inflammation in these situations. Leukocytes may also be shed into the urine during free catch collection if there is infection or inflammation within the genital tract.

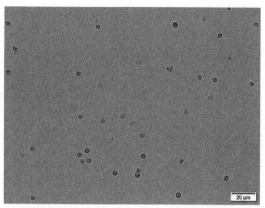

Fig. 1. Wet-mount of unstained urine sediment from an adult dog showing several erythrocytes. Erythrocytes appear as smooth, round cells that may occasionally appear crenated. Original magnification ×50.

Bacteriuria

In health, urine is sterile and thus the presence of bacteria within urine is never a normal finding (**Fig. 3**). Clinicians must consider the collection method used to help localize the source of the infection and to also assess whether iatrogenic contamination may be likely. For example, bacteriuria found within a sterile cystocentesis sample suggests infection within the bladder (cystitis) or kidneys (pyelonephritis). Conversely, bacteriuria from a free catch sample could represent kidney, bladder, or lower genital tract infection; fecal contamination could also result in iatrogenic bacteriuria. If fecal contamination is the source of bacteriuria, oftentimes the bacterial population will be pleomorphic (multiple types of cocci and rods), rather than in cases of simple urinary tract infections, which are often due to only 1 type of bacteria. In true cases of urinary tract infection, concurrent pyuria (with or without hematuria and proteinuria)

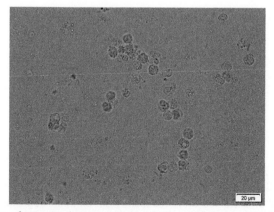

Fig. 2. Wet-mount of unstained urine sediment from an adult dog showing several leukocytes. Leukocytes are approximately twice as large as erythrocytes and contain granular-appearing cytoplasm. There are also several erythrocytes in this image, which are smaller than leukocytes. Original magnification ×50.

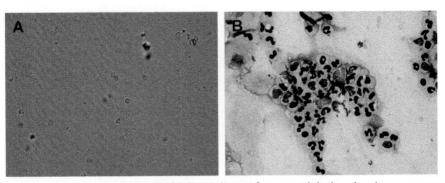

Fig. 3. (*A*) Wet-mount of unstained urine sediment from an adult dog showing numerous rod-shaped bacteria. Low numbers of erythrocytes and leukocytes are also in this image. Original magnification ×40. (*B*) Wright-Giemsa stained urine sediment from an adult dog showing segmented neutrophils with intracellular and extracellular rod-shaped bacteria. Original magnification ×50. (*Courtesy of* Reema Patel, DVM, DACVP, Antech Diagnostics, Fairfax, VA.)

is also expected and is often accompanied by appropriate clinical signs.[22] However, in some cases, bacteriuria may not be visualized, even if an infection is present. Therefore, it may be prudent to perform reflex cultures whenever leukocytes are noted on sediment examination.[23]

CRYSTALS

Crystalluria is a frequent finding in urine of dogs and cats; however, crystalluria does not always predict the presence of urolithiasis or vice versa. Although struvite (also known as triple phosphate) and calcium oxalate dihydrate crystals are common crystals (**Fig. 4**), other types of urinary crystals are highly indicative of specific underlying disease processes. Cystine crystals appear as colorless, hexagonal plates and are found in cases of hereditary cystinuria (**Fig. 5**).[22] Cystine crystalluria can predispose to urolithiasis owing to its low solubility in urine with a pH of less than 7.0.[24] Calcium

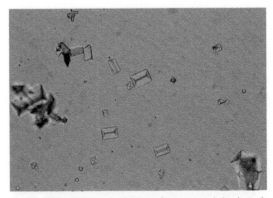

Fig. 4. Wet-mount of unstained urine sediment from an adult dog showing triple phosphate (struvite) crystals and calcium oxalate dihydrate crystals. Struvite crystals are 3-dimensional, rectangular, and colorless with a characteristic coffin lid appearance. Calcium oxalate dihydrate crystals are 3-dimensional, square, and often look similar to a closed envelope or a Maltese cross. Original magnification ×50.

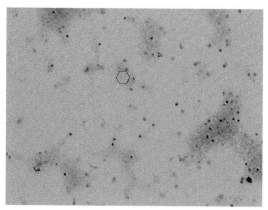

Fig. 5. Wright-Giemsa stained urine sediment from an adult dog showing a cystine crystal. These crystals appear as colorless, hexagonal plates. Original magnification ×50.

oxalate monohydrate crystals are colorless crystals, classically recognized as a picket fence shape. Their presence should create a strong suspicion for ethylene glycol toxicity, especially if clinical signs and other biochemical abnormalities supportive of ethylene glycol ingestion are observed.[22] They may also be observed in diseases resulting in hypercalciuria.[20,22] Ammonium biurate or uric acid crystals should prompt a search for underlying liver disease, but can be normal findings in Dalmatians and English Bulldogs.[21,22]

Casts

Casts are composed of a mucoprotein matrix (Tamm-Horsfall protein) that is secreted by the renal tubular epithelium. Cylindrical in appearance, they represent the shape of the tubular lumen, hence the term cast. Because they are formed by and within the tubules, casts are considered to be an indicator of renal tubular disease. However, less than 1 to 2 casts per low-power field in concentrated urine can be normal in patients without other indicators of kidney disease. Cast shedding by the tubules may be intermittent, even during active tubular disease, and the number of casts observed is not always an indicator of the type, severity, reversibility, or irreversibility of disease. Regardless, the presence of large numbers of casts upon urine sediment evaluation does indicate that there is an active pathologic process occurring within the renal tubules.[25] During urine sediment evaluation, casts are often best identified initially at low power magnification (×10 objective) and tend to be found at the edges of the wet-mount preparation, especially when only low numbers are present.

Hyaline Casts

Hyaline casts are semitransparent, colorless casts that often have blunted to rounded ends, often imparting a cylindrical appearance (**Fig. 6**). They are composed predominantly of Tamm-Horsfall mucoprotein[11,25] and usually devoid of cellular elements. These qualities can make them difficult to identify during sediment evaluation. Variable numbers of hyaline casts can be observed with either pathologic or physiological causes of proteinuria.[11,20,21] Physiological causes of hyaline casts include fever and exercise.[11] When observed in high numbers; however, glomerular protein loss should be considered, because albumin loss through the glomerulus can stimulate Tamm-Horsfall protein production and secretion from the renal tubules.[22]

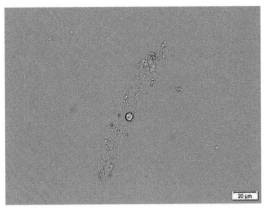

Fig. 6. Wet-mount of unstained urine sediment from an adult dog showing a single hyaline cast. These casts are rectangular and semitransparent, with indistinct borders and are composed of Tamm-Horsfall mucoprotein. Original magnification ×50.

Granular Casts

Granular casts are composed of degenerating cellular elements, in addition to mucoprotein. They have a textured appearance and may vary from clear to tan or brown in color (**Fig. 7**). The granulation may be coarse or fine in texture; finely granulated casts represent a later stage of cellular degeneration.[22] Elevated numbers of granular casts are considered an indicator of recent renal tubular injury, whereby damaged tubular epithelium slough into the lumen and partially degrade before expulsion into the urine.[21]

Waxy Casts

Waxy casts are indicative of chronic tubular disease resulting in severe urinary stasis[11,20,21] and are thought to represent the end-product of granular cast degeneration. They are denser than hyaline casts and typically have straight, blunted ends with

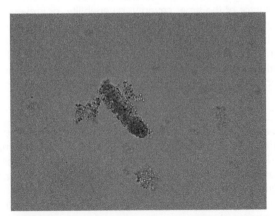

Fig. 7. Wet-mount of unstained urine sediment from an adult dog showing a granular cast. These structures are rectangular and golden-brown in color and are composed of degenerated cells and mucoprotein. Original magnification ×40.

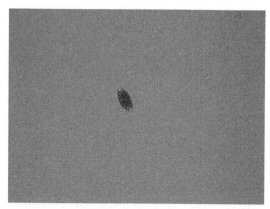

Fig. 8. Wet-mount of unstained urine sediment from an adult cat showing a single golden-brown, barrel-shaped ovum with bipolar blunted plugs, consistent with *Pearsonema* spp. Original magnification ×40. (*Courtesy of* Reema Patel, Antech Diagnostics.)

parallel sides, giving them a waxy or candlestick appearance. Waxy casts are fragile and may have fissures or cracks. They typically appear colorless to light yellow.[21]

INFECTIOUS AGENTS

Occasionally, infectious agents besides bacteria are observed during urine sediment examination. Ova from the bladder worm of dogs and cats (*Pearsonema* spp.) have bipolar plugs and an internal granular structure (**Fig. 8**). *Dioctophyma renale* ova (giant kidney worm of dogs) also have bipolar plugs but have a distinctly characteristic shell, which appears rough or pitted in appearance. Fungal infections (both primary urinary tract or systemic infections) and heartworm microfilaria (*Dirofilaria immitis*) may also be identified.[26] In some cases, these infections may be occult or can be directly correlated with the patient's presenting clinical signs. Nonetheless, the identification of any infectious agent within the urine sediment is beneficial in prompting appropriate additional diagnostic testing, if necessary, and for the commencement of appropriate therapy.

SUMMARY

The urinalysis is a diagnostic test that should not be overlooked, given the large amount of data that it can reveal about a patient's overall health status. Too often, it is avoided owing to the inconvenience of sampling, yet it is oftentimes the key to unlocking a patient's underlying disease(s). Even better yet, the urinalysis may be crucial for the early identification of numerous metabolic diseases and can allow for early intervention or prevention. The urinalysis should be considered an essential part of every diagnostic workup for ill patients, but also as essential part of the general wellness examination and should be performed regardless of the patient's age or current health status.

REFERENCES

1. Callens AJ, Bartges JW. Urinalysis. Vet Clin Small Anim 2015;45:621–37.
2. Albasan H, Lulich JP, Osborne CA, et al. Effects of storage time and temperature on pH, specific gravity, and crystal formation in urine samples from dogs and cats. J Am Vet Med Assoc 2003;222:176–9.

3. Rizzi TE, Valenciano AC, Cowell RL, et al. Initial assessment: physical characteristics. In: Rizzi TE, Valenciano AC, Cowell RL, et al, editors. Atlas of canine and feline urinalysis. 1st edition. Hoboken (NJ): Wiley-Blackwell; 2017. p. 113–9.

4. Stockham SL, Scott MA. Urinary system. In: Stockham SL, Scott MA, editors. Fundamentals of veterinary clinical pathology. 2nd edition. Ames (IA): Blackwell Publishing; 2008. p. 415–95.

5. Tvedten HW, Noren A. Comparison of a Schmidt and Haensch refractometer and an Atagon PAL-USG cat refractometer for determination of urine specific gravity in dogs and cats. Vet Clin Pathol 2014;43:63–6.

6. Trotman TK, Drobatz KJ, Hess RS. Retrospective evaluation of hyperosmolar hyperglycemia in 66 dogs (1993-2008). J Vet Emerg Crit Care (San Antonio) 2013; 23:557–64.

7. Cregar LC. Urine specific gravity. In: Wilson DA, editor. Clinical veterinary advisor: the horse. 1st edition. St Louis (MO): Elsevier-Saunders; 2012. p. 970.

8. Paquignon A, Tran G, Provost JP. Evaluation of the Clinitek 200 urinary test-strip reader in the analysis of dog and rat urines in pre-clinical toxicology studies. Lab Anim 1993;27:240–6.

9. Wilkerson MJ, Stockham SL. Assessing agreement of results of urine reagent strip assays: visual assessment versus Clinitek 100 Urine Chemistry Analyzer. In: Teaching clinical pathology, Annual meeting of the American Society for Veterinary Clinical Pathology, New Orleans, 2002, December 8–11.

10. Defontis M, Bauer N, Failing K, et al. Automated and visual analysis of commercial urinary dipsticks in dogs, cats and cattle. Res Vet Sci 2013;94:440–5.

11. Parrah JD, Moulvi BA, Gazi MA, et al. Importance of urinalysis in veterinary practice - a review. Vet World 2013;6:640–6.

12. Athanasiou LV, Katsoulos PD, Katsogiannou EG, et al. Comparison between the urine dipstick and the pH-meter to assess urine pH in sheep and dogs. Vet Clin Pathol 2018;47:284–8.

13. Thornton LA, Burchell RK, Burton SE, et al. The effect of urine concentration and pH on the growth of *Escherichia coli* in canine urine in vitro. J Vet Intern Med 2018;32:752–6.

14. Rizzi TE, Valenciano AC, Cowell RL, et al. Urine chemistry. In: Rizzi TE, Valenciano AC, Cowell RL, et al, editors. Atlas of canine and feline urinalysis. 1st edition. Hoboken (NJ): Wiley-Blackwell; 2017. p. 120–36.

15. Fletcher JM, Behrend EN, Welles EG, et al. Glucose detection and concentration estimation in feline urine samples with the Bayer Multistix and Purina Glucotest. J Feline Med Surg 2011;13:705–11.

16. Sink CA, Weinstein NM. Routine urinalysis: chemical analysis. In: Sink CA, Weinstein NM, editors. Practical veterinary urinalysis. 1st edition. Ames (IA): Wiley-Blackwell; 2012. p. 29–53.

17. Ko D-H, Jeong T-D, Kim S, et al. Influence of vitamin C on urine dipstick test results. Ann Clin Lab Sci 2015;45:391–5.

18. Vaden SL, Pressler BM, Lappin MR, et al. Effects of urinary tract inflammation and sample blood contamination on urine albumin and total protein concentrations in canine urine samples. Vet Clin Pathol 2004;33:14–9.

19. Vientos-Plotts AI, Behrend EN, Welles EG, et al. Effect of blood contamination on results of dipstick evaluation and urine protein-to-urine creatinine ratio for urine samples from dogs and cats. Am J Vet Res 2018;79:525–31.

20. Sink CA, Weinstein NM. Routine urinalysis: microscopic elements. In: Sink CA, Weinstein NM, editors. Practical veterinary urinalysis. 1st edition. Ames (IA): Wiley-Blackwell; 2012. p. 55–112.

21. Rizzi TE, Valenciano AC, Cowell RL, et al. Urine sediment. In: Rizzi TE, Valenciano AC, Cowell RL, et al, editors. Atlas of canine and feline urinalysis. 1st edition. Hoboken (NJ): Wiley-Blackwell; 2017. p. 67–179.

22. Meuten D. Laboratory evaluation and interpretation of the urinary system. In: Thrall MA, Weiser G, Allison RW, et al, editors. Veterinary hematology and clinical chemistry. 2nd edition. Ames (IA): Wiley-Blackwell; 2012. p. 323–77.

23. Tivapasi M, Hodges J, Byrne BA, et al. Diagnostic utility and cost-effectiveness of reflex bacterial culture for the detection of urinary tract infection in dogs with low urine specific gravity. Vet Clin Pathol 2009;38:337–42.

24. Hesse A, Hoffman J, Orzekowsky H, et al. Canine cystine urolithiasis: a review of 1760 submissions over 35 years (1979-2013). Can Vet J 2016;57:277–81.

25. Osborne CA, Stevens JB. Urine sediment: under the microscope. In: Osborne CA, Stevens JB, editors. Urinalysis: a clinical guide to compassionate patient care. Shawnee (KS): Bayer Corporation; 1999. p. 125–50.

26. Meyer DJ. Microscopic examination of urinary sediment. In: Raskin RE, Meyer DJ, editors. Canine and feline cytology: a color atlas and interpretation guide. 3rd edition. St Louis (MO): Elsevier; 2016. p. 295–312.

Urinary Tract Cytology

Kathryn L. Wycislo, DVM, PhD*, Tara L. Piech, DVM, MS

KEYWORDS

- Cytology • Kidney • Bladder • Nephritis • Lymphoma • Transitional cell carcinoma

KEY POINTS

- Cytology of the kidney and discrete bladder masses can be diagnostically rewarding and help to differentiate between cystic lesions, inflammation, and neoplasia.
- Traumatic catheterization is often recommended over fine needle aspiration for the sampling of bladder and urethral masses to avoid the potential for needle tract metastasis.
- Common neoplastic lesions of the urinary tract include renal carcinoma, transitional cell carcinoma of the bladder/urethra, and lymphoma.
- Cytology of urinary tract neoplasia is not always definitive and depends on various factors, such as the success of sample collection or the presence of concurrent inflammation.
- A biopsy with histopathology may be required for definitive diagnosis of benign versus malignant lesions.

INTRODUCTION

The urinary tract consists of the kidneys, ureters, bladder, and urethra. Cytologic evaluation is often performed in cases of renomegaly or when the presence of mass lesions are identified within the kidney, bladder, or urethra.[1] Cytology of the urinary tract can often help to distinguish between cystic lesions, inflammation, and neoplasia,[1] although it is often less helpful in cases of fibrosis, necrosis, interstitial nephritis, or glomerulonephritis.[2] Sampling methodology is also an important consideration when performing urinary tract cytology, as well as providing an adequate clinical history and an appropriate description of the lesion when submitting samples for evaluation by a clinical pathologist.

SAMPLING METHODS FOR URINARY TRACT CYTOLOGY
Fine Needle Aspiration

Fine needle aspirates (FNAs) of the urinary tract are frequently performed for the collection of cytologic samples from the kidneys or lesions within the urinary tract that cannot be obtained via traumatic catheterization, such as cranial bladder masses.

The authors have no conflicts of interest to disclose.
Department of Pathology and Population Medicine, Midwestern University College of Veterinary Medicine, 5715 West Utopia Road, Glendale, AZ 85308, USA
* Corresponding author.
E-mail address: kwycis@midwestern.edu

Vet Clin Small Anim 49 (2019) 247–260
https://doi.org/10.1016/j.cvsm.2018.11.002

Ultrasound-guided FNA is often recommended over blind percutaneous aspiration. Care should be taken to aspirate multiple areas of the lesion, including the lesion's center and periphery, to enhance the probability of obtaining a diagnostic sample.[2] Some lesions may contain multiple cystic or necrotic regions within or surrounding areas of solid tissue, and these various regions often appear different microscopically.

Percutaneous FNA of urethral masses or bladder masses is controversial. This controversy is due to several, albeit infrequent, reports of transitional cell carcinoma (TCC) seeding along the FNA needle tract.[3–5] Although the true incidence of needle tract metastasis secondary to TCC FNA is unknown and the exact factors that contribute to its development are poorly understood, many clinicians prefer and recommend traumatic catheterization as their collection method of choice for bladder and urethral masses. Although the authors surmise needle tract metastasis secondary to percutaneous aspiration of TCC is overall a rare event, it does not negate the possibility of its occurrence. Thus, the authors recommend that clinicians discuss the risk of needle tract metastasis secondary to percutaneous FNA with their clients and to choose the sampling method that is best suited for each individual patient.

Traumatic (Diagnostic) Catheterization

Traumatic, or diagnostic, catheterization uses a sterile catheter to disrupt tissue fragments from masslike lesions located within the bladder or urethra. It is most often used to differentiate TCC from other benign or inflammatory lesions, such as hyperplastic epithelium or cystitis. Fragments of the lesion and any accompanying fluid are collected via negative pressure into the catheter and connected syringe. Collected particulate matter can then be used to prepare squash preparations, whereas the fluid portion of the sample can be used for direct smears, cytocentrifuged preparations, or sediment examination.[6]

This collection method can be diagnostically rewarding, yielding cellular samples that are representative of the primary lesion. However, in some cases, traumatic catheterization may only result in the sampling of superficial transitional epithelial cells along the periphery of the lesion, which may lead to an inconclusive result.[2] In many instances, clinicians will have a general idea of their overall sample yield (eg, whether the amount of particulate matter obtained during traumatic catheterization was poor, adequate, or abundant). Communication of this yield to the attending clinical pathologist is important and should be included within the cytology submission form.

Touch Imprints

Touch preparations can be obtained by imprinting or rolling urinary tract biopsy specimens onto glass slides. These types of samples can be especially useful in cases where histopathologic diagnosis may be delayed, but a more expedient evaluation and diagnosis is required. If the biopsy specimen is large enough, it is first recommended to blot the cut surface of the specimen repeatedly against a paper towel until the specimen sticks to the towel. This step helps to remove superficial blood and fluid from the cut surface so that the cells of interest are more likely to exfoliate during imprinting, and blood contamination is kept to a minimum. Smaller biopsy specimens can be rolled onto glass slides with the assistance of a needle or can be used for squash preparations.[7]

Urine Sediment

In some instances, urinary tract neoplasms, such as TCC or lymphoma, may exfoliate into the urine, allowing for neoplastic cells to be identified during urine sediment examination. However, clinicians should be aware that cytologic examination of the urine sediment for the presence of urinary tract neoplasia is often not definitively conclusive and may require additional sampling by one of the techniques mentioned previously.[2]

CYTOLOGY SUBMISSION RECOMMENDATIONS FOR URINARY TRACT LESIONS

Similar to all other types of cytologic evaluations, the attending clinical pathologist must use experience and data-driven information to form accurate (and to avoid inaccurate) interpretations when evaluating FNAs from the urinary tract. Signalment, location, and description of the lesion(s), along with a brief but relevant clinical history are all necessary requirements for a cytologist to make the best interpretation of the sample they have been provided, and to facilitate the generation of helpful comments for the submitting clinician (**Box 1**).

NORMAL KIDNEY CYTOLOGY

In general, aspirates of normal kidney parenchyma are typically of low nucleated cellularity, consisting primarily of renal tubular epithelial cells and occasional glomerular tufts (**Fig. 1A**). Blood contamination is a frequent and expected finding, given the high vascularity of the kidney. Renal tubular epithelial cells are visualized as monomorphic round to cuboidal cells with moderate amounts of basophilic cytoplasm and a single, round, centrally placed nucleus. They may be found individually, in small

---

Box 1
Recommendations on patient and lesion information for urinary tract cytology samples.

- Patient signalment
  - Breed, age, and neuter status

- Location and size of the lesion(s) identified
  - Bilateral or unilateral
  - Single or multifocal
  - Approximate size (centimeters, inches, or relative size to common objects)
  - Other relevant descriptors as deemed appropriate
    - Discrete versus diffuse lesion
    - Localized versus invasive
    - Location within the bladder
      - Body versus trigone
      - Cranioventral versus craniodorsal
    - Location within the kidney, if a discrete lesion
      - Cranial or caudal pole

- Clinician's opinion of sample yield
  - Poorly or readily exfoliative?

- Clinical signs associated with lesion(s)
  - Abnormalities in micturition (dysuria, stranguria, pollakiuria, etc.)
  - Abnormal urinalysis findings (hematuria, inflammation, etc.)

- Relevant clinical history
  - Examples
    - History of chronic, recurrent urinary tract infections
    - History of cystic calculi
    - Previous history of fungal infection or other infectious agents
    - Other organ systems currently affected

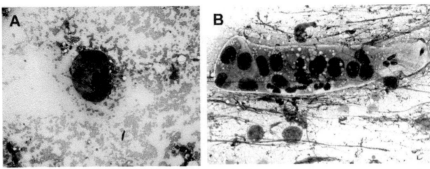

Fig. 1. (A) Renal aspirate from an adult cat showing a glomerular tuft (original magnification ×10 obj.; stain: Wright-Giemsa). (B) Renal aspirate from an adult cat showing a renal tubule with associated neutrophils (original magnification ×60 obj.; stain: Wright-Giemsa). (*Courtesy of* Natalie Hoepp, University of Pennsylvania School of Veterinary Medicine, Philadelphia, PA.)

cohesive sheets, or in tubular arrangements (**Fig. 1**B).[2,6] Occasionally, aspirates may yield tubular epithelial cells that contain black granular cytoplasmic pigment,[2,6] consistent with aspiration of the ascending loop of Henle or distal tubules.[2] In feline kidney samples, renal tubular epithelial cells often contain lipid, which is observed as distinct, clear cytoplasmic vacuoles.[6] Minimal numbers of inflammatory cells and minimal cellular pleomorphism should be observed.

THE KIDNEY: NONNEOPLASTIC AND INFLAMMATORY LESIONS

Various nonneoplastic lesions can affect the kidney, including cysts, amyloidosis, and inflammation (nephritis). In these authors' experience, cytology of the kidney is often most rewarding in cases of inflammation, which can be due to both infectious and noninfectious causes.

Renal Cysts

Renal cysts can be congenital or acquired, as well as single or multiple. Grossly, renal cysts contain clear or yellow tinted fluid.[2] Cytologically, they contain a stippled to densely amorphous eosinophilic background and are typically of low nucleated cellularity. Nucleated cells often consist primarily of macrophages.[2] It is important to note that if neoplasia is clinically suspected, FNA of a more solid tissue area of the mass should be performed, because samples interpreted as cystic lesions may not be entirely representative of the true underlying pathology.[2] Renal adenocarcinomas may have cystic regions that mimic the appearance of benign cysts on cytology.[6] A dominantly inherited condition, renal cystadenocarcinoma and nodular dermatofibrosis, has been well-characterized in German Shepherd dogs. Dogs with this condition present with multiple firm cutaneous nodules and often bilateral, multiple renal cysts and renal cystadenocarcinoma.[8] Renal cystadenocarcinoma and nodular dermatofibrosis is caused by a mutation in folliculin, a tumor suppressor gene.[9]

Renal Amyloidosis

Renal amyloid deposition may be organ limited or disseminated and related to systemic amyloidosis.[10] Familial amyloidosis is recognized in Chinese Shar-Pei dogs as well as Abyssinian cats and is generally classified as a subtype of reactive amyloidosis.[10] In reactive amyloidosis, amyloid is composed of the acute phase protein serum amyloid A.[10] Other causes of reactive amyloidosis include idiopathic causes, infectious disease, chronic inflammation, or neoplasia.[10] Cytologically, amyloid appears as undulous, glassy swirls of amorphous eosinophilic material that may be observed in close association with glomeruli or renal tubular epithelial cells.[2] This material may be mistaken for collagen or extracellular matrix, which both appear similar cytologically. Amyloid is classically apple-green birefringent when stained with Congo red and examined under polarized light.[2]

Renal Crystals

Crystals are rarely observed in kidney FNAs; however, both calcium oxalate monohydrate crystals and melamine–cyanuric acid crystals have been reported.[2] Melamine–cyanuric acid crystals have been associated with ingestion of contaminated pet food, and appear as round to dumbbell-shaped, green to yellow striated crystals[2] associated with the distal tubules and collecting ducts.[11] Calcium oxalate monohydrate crystals can be associated with ethylene glycol toxicosis or can be an incidental finding. These crystals appear as elongated, hexagonal, colorless, picket fence-shaped crystals that may be associated with proximal renal tubular epithelial cells.[12] Both types of crystals are birefringent when viewed under polarized light.[1]

Renal Inflammation

Nephritis refers to inflammation within the kidney, which may result from ascending lower urinary tract infections or from disseminated infectious or noninfectious diseases.[2] FNAs from kidney inflammation are typically highly cellular. As discussed elsewhere in this article, kidney FNAs often contain a significant amount of blood contamination with associated leukocytes. Therefore, the clinical pathologist must carefully evaluate the proportions of inflammatory cells present in kidney FNAs within the context of blood contamination, to accurately determine whether leukocytes are truly increased in number.

As with other lesions throughout the body, the type of inflammation within kidney FNAs can help to narrow down the list of possible causes or etiologic agents. For instance, suppurative nephritis is often associated with a bacterial or possibly immune-mediated etiology, whereas pyogranulomatous or granulomatous nephritis can be associated with fungal, protozoal, algal, or higher order bacterial etiologies. In lesions that contain severe or overwhelming inflammation, neutrophils may exhibit a degenerate morphology, consisting of pale, swollen nuclei. Macrophages may appear activated (increased size and amount of vacuolated cytoplasm) or be found in epithelioid sheets.[2]

Reported pyogranulomatous or granulomatous nephritis etiologies include feline infectious peritonitis, *Mycobacterium* spp., and systemic fungal or protozoal infections (such as *Aspergillus* spp. and *Leishmania* spp., respectively; **Fig. 2**). Many infectious agents can be readily identified on cytology; however, culture and/or polymerase chain reaction are more sensitive methods by which to detect these organisms if no specific agent is identified.[2]

Lymphocytic–plasmacytic inflammation is often associated with interstitial nephritis and chronic kidney disease; however, the cause of these conditions is usually not apparent on kidney cytology[6] and biopsy with histopathology is necessary to differentiate between certain disease processes, such as interstitial nephritis or glomerulonephritis. Lymphocytic–plasmacytic inflammation can be distinguished from lymphoma by a predominance of small, mature lymphocytes and plasma cells. In contrast, most

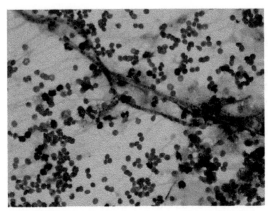

Fig. 2. Fungal nephritis. Renal aspirate from a young male castrated German Shepherd dog with bilateral renomegaly. Suppurative inflammation is observed, along with elongated, basophilic, septate fungal hyphae. The hyphae are morphologically consistent with *Aspergillus* spp. or *Penicillium* spp., but further diagnostic testing was not pursued in this case (original magnification ×50 obj.; stain: Wright-Giemsa).

cases of renal lymphoma are predominated by large monomorphic lymphocytes, which often have immature chromatin and prominent nucleoli.

THE KIDNEY: NEOPLASTIC LESIONS

Neoplasms of the kidney may be primary or metastatic (secondary). Primary renal neoplasia is rare in both dogs and cats, and accounts for approximately 1% of all canine neoplasms and 1% to 2% of all feline neoplasms.[1] Of all kidney tumors, approximately 32% are primary in dogs compared with 12% in cats.[9] The vast majority of primary kidney neoplasms in both species consist of malignant epithelial tumors, such as renal carcinoma or adenocarcinoma, which may be unilateral or bilateral, as well as single or multiple.[2] Of primary kidney neoplasms, renal carcinoma accounts for approximately 75% of all canine neoplasms and 77% of all feline neoplasms. Other carcinomas, such as TCC, squamous cell carcinoma, and metastatic carcinoma of the kidney are less common than renal carcinoma.[6]

Renal lymphoma in both species is more commonly associated with metastatic disease rather than primary neoplasia. The reported incidence of renal lymphoma is much higher in cats (88% of all secondary renal neoplasms) compared with dogs (23% of all secondary renal neoplasms). Other reported secondary renal neoplasms consist of mesenchymal tumors, such as hemangiosarcoma, which have a higher incidence in dogs compared with cats.[9] With the exception of sarcomas, many renal neoplasms are highly exfoliative, and kidney FNA is often diagnostically rewarding in these cases, particularly if discrete masses or renomegaly are noted on abdominal imaging.

Renal Carcinoma

Renal carcinoma samples are often of high nucleated cellularity and contain variably cohesive aggregates of polygonal to rounded epithelial cells.[2] Well-differentiated renal carcinomas can be difficult to distinguish from reactive epithelial hyperplasia, particularly if concurrent inflammation is present, because the epithelial cells may display only minimal anisocytosis and anisokaryosis (**Fig. 3**). In these cases, biopsy with histopathologic evaluation is often necessary to distinguish between reactive epithelium

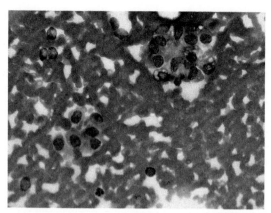

Fig. 3. Well-differentiated renal carcinoma. Renal mass from a 14-year-old cat. Several small clusters of polygonal-shaped epithelial cells are present and display only minimal pleomorphism. These cells have a moderate amount of basophilic cytoplasm and round nuclei with variably distinct nucleoli (original magnification ×50 obj.; stain: Wright-Giemsa).

and neoplastic epithelium. In contrast, poorly differentiated renal carcinomas often display moderate to marked anisocytosis and anisokaryosis, with variable nuclear to cytoplasmic (N:C) ratios and immature chromatin (**Fig. 4**A).[2] Rarely, renal carcinomas have also been shown to exhibit basement membrane production (hyaline globules) by the neoplastic cells (**Fig. 4**B).[13]

Nephroblastoma

Nephroblastomas typically present as a unilateral, single renal or spinal mass that affects young dogs and cats and arises from embryonic metanephric blastema.[9] These neoplasms are rare, and only constitute up to 5% of primary kidney neoplasms in small animals.[9] They contain 3 distinct cell populations, including epithelial, blastemal,

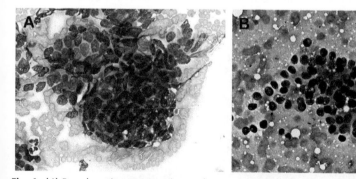

Fig. 4. (*A*) Renal carcinoma. Renal mass from a 2-year-old cat. Dense cohesive aggregates of epithelium are poorly-differentiated with large nuclei and prominent nucleoli (original magnification ×50 obj.; stain: Wright-Giemsa). (*B*) Basement membrane production, renal carcinoma. Renal mass from an adult dog. Aggregates of epithelial cells have indistinct borders and high nuclear to cytoplasmic ratios. Amorphous extracellular eosinophilic material is observed among the clusters, which is suspected to represent basement membrane production by neoplastic cells (original magnification ×60 obj.; stain: Wright-Giemsa). (*Courtesy of* [A] Khush Banajee, Antech Diagnostics, Mount Laurel, NJ; and [B] Tricia Bisby, Antech Diagnostics, Oak Brook, IL, and Reema Patel, Antech Diagnostics, Fairfax, VA.)

and mesenchymal cells.[9] Histologically, on immunohistochemistry these neoplasms will exhibit cytokeratin as well as vimentin positivity for the epithelial and mesenchymal components, respectively.[2] Immunohistochemical expression of Wilms' tumor gene product also helps to confirm nephroblastoma.[1] The epithelial cells are often highly exfoliative and are present in loosely cohesive clusters or sheets. They often display minimal cytologic criteria of malignancy, with indistinct nucleoli, finely stippled chromatin, and mild anisocytosis and anisokaryosis.[2] The cells typically have high N:C ratios, with scant amounts of lightly basophilic cytoplasm and can mimic the cytologic appearance of round cell neoplasms (especially lymphoma) or neuroendocrine neoplasms (**Fig. 5**).[2,6] Blastemal cells may also be present cytologically and appear as small, condensed cells with high N:C ratios and indistinct cytoplasmic borders.[14] The mesenchymal component is typically poorly exfoliative.[14]

Renal Lymphoma

Renal lymphoma may originate as a primary or metastatic neoplasm and is more common in cats than in dogs[2]; in fact, it is the most common kidney neoplasm in felines.[15] Older cats (>10 years of age) are predisposed and median survival times for feline renal lymphoma are significantly shorter compared with lymphoma in other anatomic locations. Most feline lymphomas are of B-cell origin.[16]

Ultrasonographically, renal lymphoma appears similar in both dogs and cats, and consists of renomegaly with increased hypoechogenicity of the renal cortex and focal or multifocal diffusely hypoechoic lesions throughout the renal parenchyma.[15] Most lymphomatous lesions in dogs are also hypoechoic, but hyperechogenicity has also been reported.[17] FNAs of renal lymphoma often exfoliate readily, which usually results in high cellularity.[6] Samples typically consist of sheets of monomorphic large lymphocytes that have high N:C ratios with a scant amount of basophilic cytoplasm (**Fig. 6**A). Fine azurophilic granules or small clear vacuoles may be present within the cytoplasm; these findings should raise suspicion for granular lymphoma or T-cell lymphoma, respectively. Nucleoli are often prominent and may exhibit variation in size, shape, and number. Because neoplastic lymphocytes are often fragile and prone to disruption during sample collection, the samples may contain numerous bare nuclei from ruptured cells (smudge cells).

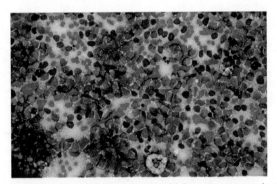

Fig. 5. Nephroblastoma. Renal mass from a 1-year-old dog. Numerous clusters and sheets of round cells with high nuclear to cytoplasmic ratios and numerous cytoplasmic vacuoles are observed. Cytologically, this could be easily confused with lymphoma, but the patient's young age makes nephroblastoma an important differential to consider (original magnification ×20 obj.; stain: Wright-Giemsa). (*Courtesy of* John Bjorneby, Antech Diagnostics, Carlsbad, CA.)

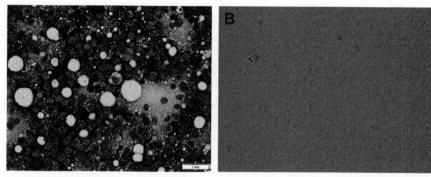

Fig. 6. (*A*) Renal lymphoma. Renal mass from an adult cat showing a monomorphic popu-lation of large lymphocytes with high nuclear to cytoplasmic ratios and frequent cyto-plasmic vacuolation, consistent with lymphoma (original magnification ×60 obj.; stain: Wright-Giemsa. (*B*) Urine sediment, renal lymphoma. Wet mount of unstained urine sedi-ment from an adult cat. Large nucleated cells with high nuclear to cytoplasmic ratios and prominent nucleoli are appreciated even on wet mount, along with a few erythrocytes. A stained urine sediment confirmed the presence of lymphoblasts (original magnification ×50 obj.). (*Courtesy of* [A] Natalie Hoepp, University of Pennsylvania School of Veterinary Medicine, Philadelphia, PA; and [B] Reema Patel, Antech Diagnostics, Fairfax, VA.)

If a definitive cytologic diagnosis of lymphoma cannot be achieved, further advanced diagnostics are recommended. Other than biopsy with histopathologic evaluation, polymerase chain reaction for antigen receptor rearrangement or flow cytometry may be pursued. Polymerase chain reaction for antigen receptor rearrange-ment can help to differentiate between reactive lymphoid hyperplasia and lymphoma, and can be performed on stained or unstained cytology slides. Flow cytometry is often most helpful for phenotyping a previously diagnosed lymphoma. Less commonly, renal lymphoma may be detected upon microscopic examination of urine sediment by the presence of lymphoblasts (**Fig. 6**B). Stained cytocentrifuged preparations of urine sediment often aid in the diagnosis.

Renal Sarcoma

Renal sarcomas may also be primary (originating from renal parenchymal elements such as vessels) or metastatic[2] and are relatively uncommon. Mesenchymal neo-plasms constitute roughly 25% of primary kidney tumors in dogs.[9] Aspirates are often poorly exfoliative and usually consist of individual and variably sized aggregates of spindle cells that have variable N:C ratios, with moderate amounts of basophilic, wispy to stellate cytoplasm, and variably prominent nucleoli.[2] Some reported renal sarcomas include fibrosarcoma,[6] hemangiosarcoma, extraskeletal osteosarcoma (**Fig. 7**), chon-drosarcoma,[18] and histiocytic sarcoma.[19] Alkaline phosphatase staining of previously unstained cytology slides can help to differentiate between osteosarcomas and other sarcomas, because osteoblasts will display alkaline phosphatase positivity.[20]

THE BLADDER: NONNEOPLASTIC AND INFLAMMATORY LESIONS

Most cases of bladder inflammation (cystitis) can be presumptively diagnosed through the identification of increased numbers of leukocytes (with or without accompanying bacteriuria) during urine sediment examination, especially when correlated with clin-ical history and appropriate physical examination findings.[6] Although chronic cystitis may result in transitional cell hyperplasia and a thickened bladder wall,[6] nonneoplastic

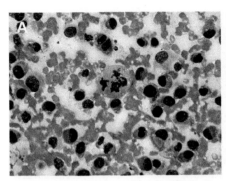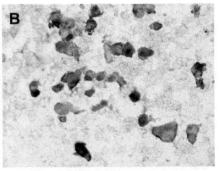

Fig. 7. Osteosarcoma. (*A*) Renal aspirate from an adult dog with multifocal heterogeneous lesions on abdominal ultrasound examination. Numerous individualized, rounded, plasmacytoid osteoblasts are shown that display moderate to marked anisocytosis and anisokaryosis (original magnification ×60 obj.; stain: Wright-Giemsa). (*B*) BCIP-NBT staining for alkaline phosphatase activity was positive, consistent with a diagnosis of osteosarcoma (original magnification ×60 obj).

and inflammatory lesions within the bladder can sometimes result in discrete, masslike lesions that are amenable to FNA. Diagnosis of cystitis via urine sediment examination is covered in Tara L. Piech and Kathryn L. Wycislo's article, "Importance of Urinalysis," elsewhere in this issue.

Polypoid Cystitis

Polypoid cystitis is a nonneoplastic inflammatory condition characterized by the formation of one to multiple masslike proliferations within the bladder.[9] It is most frequently reported in dogs with a history of hematuria.[21–23] Patients may also present with a history of recurrent urinary tract infection or cystic calculi.[21] The masslike proliferations are composed of hyperplastic transitional cells and variable amounts of inflammation, hence the term cystitis.[9,21] Grossly, polypoid cystitis lesions may be ulcerated, hemorrhagic, and difficult to differentiate from TCC; however, polypoid cystitis is treated differently and has a better prognosis than TCC.[9,24] Thus, visualization of any masslike lesion within the bladder, whether single or multiple in nature, is a reasonable indication for further diagnostics such as cytology.

Cytologically, a differential of polypoid cystitis should be considered whenever a masslike lesion yields transitional epithelial cells that display mild to moderate cellular atypia (**Fig. 8**). Concurrent inflammation may also be present.[6] The hyperplastic transitional epithelial cells may exfoliate in large clusters or sheets. In lesions that display mild pleomorphism, the transitional cells are often observed as round to cuboidal cells with distinct cellular junctions, moderate amounts of basophilic cytoplasm, and single round nuclei with coarse chromatin and inconspicuous nucleoli.[2] When moderate pleomorphism is observed, cytologic findings may include increased basophilia, binucleation, and more prominent anisocytosis. These features may raise a cytologist's concern for a well-differentiated TCC; however, the nuclear criteria of malignancy should not be a frequent finding in cases of hyperplasia.[6]

The differentiation of polypoid cystitis from other nonneoplastic lesions within the bladder cannot be determined definitively by cytology alone, and cytologic interpretations will typically suggest either hyperplastic lesions, polypoid or polyp lesions, or a papilloma as potential differentials.[2] Biopsy is also often needed to rule out underlying malignancy, given the potential for both polypoid cystitis and TCC to occur concurrently, and in cases with significant pleomorphism that are also inflamed.[6]

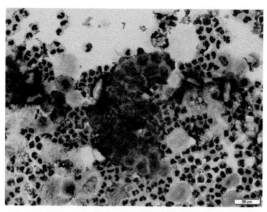

Fig. 8. Polypoid cystitis. Traumatic catheterization sample from an adult dog with an apical bladder mass, hematuria, and cystic calculi. A sheet of hyperplastic transitional epithelial cells display moderate atypia and are surrounded by numerous degenerate neutrophils and bacterial cocci. Histopathology confirmed this nonneoplastic condition (original magnification ×50 obj.; stain: Wright-Giemsa).

Polyp

Bladder polyps are singular lesions attached to a stalk that are histologically similar to polypoid cystitis lesions.[9] Cytologic samples from a polyp should contain hyperplastic transitional epithelium that do not display marked cytologic criteria of malignancy, similar to the expected cytologic findings in polypoid cystitis and papilloma, thus necessitating histopathology for definitive determination.[2]

Papilloma

Papillomas that arise from the urinary bladder are differentiated histologically from polyploid lesions based on an absence of inflammatory cells and the presence of focal papillary projections of transitional cells. They are considered uncommon lesions, comprising only about 2% of reported canine bladder tumors.[9] When evaluated cytologically, papillomas may display more nuclear pleomorphism, such as increased anisokaryosis and a variable N:C ratio, than the hyperplastic transitional cells observed in polypoid cystitis and polyps.[2]

THE BLADDER: NEOPLASTIC LESIONS

TCC is by far the most common malignancy of the urinary bladder and urethra in both cats and dogs, ranging anywhere from 75% to 90% of the bladder tumors reported in these species. Benign epithelial tumors of the bladder are exceedingly rare. The remainder of bladder tumors are composed predominantly of mesenchymal tumors of either smooth muscle, skeletal muscle, fibrocyte, or endothelial cell origin, which may be either benign or malignant in nature.[9] Round cell neoplasms, such as lymphoma, have also been reported in the bladder.[25,26]

Transitional Cell Carcinoma

Most commonly arising from the trigone area of the bladder in dogs,[9,24,27] TCC is an aggressive neoplasm that often presents with nonspecific signs related to urinary tract disease (such as hematuria, pollakiuria, and cystitis).[27,28] In some cases, the primary lesion may be large enough to partially or completely obstruct urinary outflow. Concurrent involvement of the urethra and/or prostate are common.[29] TCC in cats may be

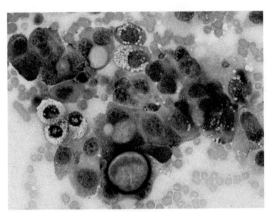

Fig. 9. Transitional cell carcinoma. Bladder mass aspirate (trigone region) from an adult dog. Polygonal to rounded epithelial cells display marked anisocytosis and anisokaryosis, as well as binucleation. Some cells contain large magenta inclusions consistent with Melamed-Wolinska bodies. (original magnification ×50 obj.; stain: Wright-Giemsa).

found within the trigone (approximately 50% of cases), the ventral wall, fundus, or neck of the bladder.[9] Grossly, TCC may present as one to multiple lesions with a thickened bladder wall and/or papillary projections into the bladder wall; yet, it may also mimic the appearance of other bladder neoplasms, necessitating either cytologic or histologic diagnosis.[9,24]

TCC cytology is often diagnostic, except in cases of well-differentiated TCC (displaying minimal pleomorphism) or when sampling only achieves collection of surrounding hyperplastic epithelium. Marked concurrent inflammation within the sample may also make a diagnosis of TCC equivocal, because hyperplastic or dysplastic epithelium can often mimic the cytologic appearance of neoplastic epithelium. However, many TCCs are highly pleomorphic and display marked cytologic criteria of malignancy. Cells often exfoliate individually or in cohesive clusters with distinct cytoplasmic junctions. TCCs also commonly contain single to multiple bright magenta cytoplasmic vacuoles, called Melamed–Wolinska bodies, which are a unique feature of TCC (**Fig. 9**).[9,30] The vacuoles stain periodic acid–Schiff and uroplakin positive and may impart a signet ring appearance to the cell. Additionally, identification of Melamed–Wolinska bodies in carcinomas outside the urinary tract can help to raise suspicion for metastatic TCC.[9]

SUMMARY

Clinicians should consider performing urinary tract cytology whenever a patient presents with abnormalities within the urinary tract that are conducive to cytologic sampling. Although not all cytologic samples from the urinary tract will result in a definitive diagnosis and some may require histopathologic follow-up, urinary tract cytology of many kidney and bladder lesions (particularly TCC, lymphoma, and inflammatory/infectious conditions) are often highly informative. In these instances, urinary tract cytology may prevent the need for more invasive procedures and allow appropriate therapy to rapidly commence.

REFERENCES

1. Ewing PJ, Meinkoth JH, Cowell RL, et al. The kidneys. In: Valenciano AC, Cowell RL, editors. Cowell and Tyler's diagnostic cytology and hematology of the dog and cat. 4th edition. St Louis (MO): Elsevier Mosby; 2014. p. 387–401.

2. Borjesson DL, DeJong K. Urinary tract. In: Raskin RE, Meyer DJ, editors. Canine and feline cytology: a color atlas and interpretation guide. 3rd edition. St Louis (MO): Elsevier; 2016. p. 284–94.

3. Nyland TG, Wallack ST, Wisner ER. Needle-tract implantation following US-guided fine-needle aspiration biopsy of transitional cell carcinoma of the bladder, urethra, and prostate. Vet Radiol Ultrasound 2002;43(1):50–3.

4. Moore AR, Coffey E, Leavell SE, et al. Canine bicavitary carcinomatosis with transient needle tract metastasis diagnosed by multiplex immunocytochemistry. Vet Clin Pathol 2016;45:495–500.

5. Klopfleisch R, Sperling C, Kershaw O, et al. Does the taking of biopsies affect the metastatic potential of tumors? A systemic review of reports on veterinary and human cases and animal models. Vet J 2011;190:e31–42.

6. Webb JL. Renal cytology and urinalysis. In: Barger AM, MacNeill AL, editors. Small animal cytologic diagnosis. 1st edition. Boca Raton (FL): Taylor & Francis Group; 2017. p. 357–63.

7. Meyer DJ. Acquisition and management of cytology specimens. In: Raskin RE, Meyer DJ, editors. Canine and feline cytology: a color atlas and interpretation guide. 3rd edition. St Louis (MO): Elsevier; 2016. p. 8.

8. Bonsdorff TB, Jansen JH, Thomassen RF, et al. Loss of heterozygosity at the FLCN locus in early renal cystic lesions in dogs with renal cystadenocarcinoma and nodular dermatofibrosis. Mamm Genome 2009;20:315–20.

9. Meuten DJ, Meuten TLK. Tumors of the urinary system. In: Meuten DJ, editor. Tumors in domestic animals. 5th edition. Ames (IA): John Wiley & Sons, Inc.; 2017. p. 632–88.

10. Segev G, Cowgill LD, Jessen S, et al. Renal amyloidosis in dogs: a retrospective study of 91 cases with comparison of the disease between Shar-Pei and non-Shar-Pei dogs. J Vet Intern Med 2012;26:259–68.

11. Brown CA, Jeong K-S, Poppenga RH, et al. Outbreaks of renal failure associated with melamine and cyanuric acid in dogs and cats in 2004 and 2007. J Vet Diagn Invest 2007;19:525–31.

12. Barigye R, Mostrom M, Dyer NW, et al. Ethylene glycol toxicosis in adult beef cattle fed contaminated feeds. Can Vet J 2008;49(10):1018–20.

13. Collicutt NB, Garner BC, Brown C, et al. What is your diagnosis? Renal mass in a dog. Vet Clin Pathol 2013;42(3):389–90.

14. Michael HT, Sharkey LC, Kovi RC, et al. Pathology in practice. J Am Vet Med Assoc 2013;242(4):471–3.

15. Debruyn K, Haers K, Combes A, et al. Ultrasonography of the feline kidney. J Feline Med Surg 2012;14:794–803.

16. Collette SA, Allstadt SD, Chon EM, et al. Treatment of feline intermediate to high-grade lymphoma with a modified university of Wisconsin–Madison protocol: 119 cases (2004–2012). Vet Comp Oncol 2016;13:136–46.

17. Taylor AJ, Lara-Garcia A, Benigni L. Ultrasonographic characteristics of canine renal lymphoma. Vet Radiol Ultrasound 2014;55(4):441–6.

18. Hahn KA, McGavin MD, Adams WH. Bilateral renal metastases of nasal chondrosarcoma in a dog. Vet Pathol 1997;34:352–5.

19. Affolter VK, Moore PF. Localized and disseminated histiocytic sarcoma of dendritic cell origin in dogs. Vet Pathol 2002;39:74–83.

20. Barger A, Graca R, Bailey K, et al. Use of alkaline phosphatase staining to differentiate canine osteosarcoma from other vimentin-positive tumors. Vet Pathol 2005;42:161–5.

21. Martinez I, Mattoon JS, Eaton KA, et al. Polypoid cystitis in 17 dogs (1978-2001). J Vet Intern Med 2003;17:499–509.
22. Lopez J, Norman BC. Ultrasound-guided urinary catheter bladder biopsy through a urinary catheter in a bitch. J Am Anim Hosp Assoc 2014;50:414–6.
23. Takiguchi M, Inaba A. Diagnostic ultrasound of polypoid cystitis in dogs. J Vet Med Sci 2005;67:57–61.
24. Knapp DW, McMillan SK. Tumors of the urinary system. In: Withrow SJ, Vail DM, Page RL, editors. Withrow and MacEwen's small animal clinical oncology. 5th edition. St Louis (MO): Saunders; 2012. p. 574–6.
25. Maiolino P, DeVico G. Primary epitheliotropic T-cell lymphoma of the urinary bladder in a dog. Vet Pathol 2000;37:184–6.
26. Benigni L, Lamb CR, Corzo-Menendez N, et al. Lymphoma affecting the urinary bladder in three dogs and a cat. Vet Radiol Ultrasound 2006;47:592–6.
27. Mutsaers AJ, Widmer WR, Knapp DW. Canine transitional cell carcinoma. J Vet Intern Med 2003;17:136–44.
28. Norris AM, Laing EJ, Valli VE, et al. Canine bladder and urethral tumors: a retrospective study of 115 cases (1908-1985). J Vet Intern Med 1992;6:145–53.
29. Knapp DW, Glickman NW, Denicola DB, et al. Naturally-occurring canine transitional cell carcinoma of the urinary bladder: a relevant model of human invasive bladder cancer. Urol Oncol 2000;5:47–59.
30. Webb KL, Marks Stowe D, DeVanna J, et al. Pathology in practice. Transitional cell carcinoma. J Am Vet Med Assoc 2015;247:1249–51.

Diagnostic Imaging of the Urinary Tract

Nathalie Rademacher, Dr Med Vet

KEYWORDS

• Imaging • Urinary tract • Ultrasonography • CT • Abdomen • Contrast studies

KEY POINTS

- Imaging of patients with urinary tract diseases is an integral part of the diagnostic work-up, and multiple imaging modalities are available.
- Survey radiographs are still being used as a screening method because of the ease of the modality.
- Ultrasonography is the main modality of choice for an initial work-up, followed by contrast radiology, whereas now excretory urography computed tomography is the modality of choice for evaluation for ectopic ureters.

INTRODUCTION

Imaging of patients with urinary tract diseases is an integral part of the diagnostic work-up, and multiple imaging modalities are available. It is important to select the appropriate modality based on the clinical presentation and question.[1–4] Radiographs are, to this date, the classic first step and screening method in the work-up of patients with urinary signs because of the availability, ease of acquisition, and low cost. Ultrasonography has become the modality of choice after survey radiographs because of the ability of internal assessment of the kidneys and urinary bladder and ease of assessment in the hands of experienced ultrasonographers.[5] Limitations of ultrasonography include the inability to evaluate kidneys in some large or obese dogs or in dogs with excessive bowel gas. In addition, the integrity of the urinary tract in cases of trauma cannot be assessed with ultrasonography. In these cases, and for the evaluation for ectopic ureters, urinary contrast studies are the method of choice.[4] Commonly used urinary tract contrast procedures in small animals include excretory urography (EU), also known as intravenous pyelogram (IVP), retrograde urethrography, and retrograde cystography. A short overview of the different methods is given here, with a short summary on contrast agents in **Box 1**. Computed tomography (CT) EU (CTEU) is now the method of choice in the evaluation of ectopic ureters and

Section of Radiology, Veterinary Clinical Sciences, School of Veterinary Medicine, Louisiana State University, Baton Rouge, LA, USA
E-mail address: nrademac@lsu.edu

Vet Clin Small Anim 49 (2019) 261–286
https://doi.org/10.1016/j.cvsm.2018.10.006
0195-5616/19/© 2018 Elsevier Inc. All rights reserved.

vetsmall.theclinics.com

Box 1
Contrast agents used in veterinary medicine

Radiolucent (negative) contrast agents:

- Primarily used for double-contrast or negative contrast cystograms

- Room air is used most frequently but carbon dioxide and nitrous oxide are safer negative contrast media because their increased solubility makes air embolization less likely. A source of carbon dioxide is pressurized canisters. Never attached directly to the patient. Always fill a syringe first, and then inject it from an atmospheric pressure syringe.

Radiopaque (positive) contrast agents:

- Ionic iodides: these agents are water-soluble triiodinated benzoic acid derivatives. Ionic iodides are either diatrizoate or iothalamate combined with sodium or meglumine. It is best not to use pure sodium contrast in patients with congestive heart failure.

- Nonionic iodides: these contrast agents are the most widespread and commonly used agents for any contrast procedure because of decreased cost and increased safety to the patient, especially in high-risk patients. The main advantage of nonionized iodides is that they do not dissolve into positive and negative ions when placed into solutions such as blood or cerebrospinal fluid because of lower osmolarity.[30,31]

---

its importance is likely to increase in the coming years.[6–9] The following represents an overview of the different modalities available for the different areas of the urinary tract.

KIDNEYS AND URETERS

Three (left and right lateral, and ventrodorsal [VD]) radiographic views are needed for complete evaluation of the abdomen.[1] Right lateral radiographs provide more longitudinal separation between the right and left kidneys. The kidneys are located in the retroperitoneal space and are generally surrounded by fat. In very thin animals with little retroperitoneal fat or in cases of retroperitoneal fluid collection (urine or blood from trauma), the kidneys are more difficult to visualize (**Fig. 1**). In the dog, the cranial pole of the right kidney is approximately at the level of T13 to L1 and at L2 to L3 for the cranial pole of the left kidney. The cranial pole of the right kidney is often difficult to see

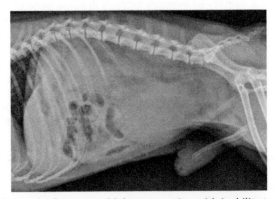

Fig. 1. Lateral radiograph of a 4-year-old dog presenting with inability to urinate. Note the decreased detail in the retroperitoneal space, border effacing the kidneys, colon, and dorsal border of the urinary bladder. The retroperitoneal effusion in this case was the result of ureteral obstruction.

because it silhouettes with the caudate lobe of the liver. Normal dogs have kidney lengths 2.5 to 3.5 times the length of the body of L2, measured on the VD view. In the cat, the right kidney is located between L1 and L4 and the left kidney between L2 and L5. The normal cat kidney size ranges from 2 to 3 times the length of the body of L2. Cat kidneys are very mobile, especially the left. Both kidneys should have a smooth margin and be of similar size and shape. Variations in size, shape, and opacity may aid in a diagnosis of kidney disease (**Fig. 2, Tables 1** and **2**). Variation in location may be secondary to kidney masses (**Fig. 3**A, B), adrenomegaly (lateral and caudal displacement; **Fig. 3**C, D), hepatomegaly (caudal displacement), gastric dilatation (caudal displacement), and ovarian masses (lateral and cranial displacement). Ultrasonography is the method of choice to evaluate the urinary tract because of the ability to assess internal architecture and vascularity. Ultrasonography findings are often non–disease specific; however differentiation of acute versus chronic kidney changes (**Fig. 4**), mass lesions (**Fig. 5**), cysts (see **Fig. 4B; Fig. 6**), mineralization (**Figs. 4C** and **7**), and alterations of the collecting system and ureters (**Fig. 8**) is possible.[5]

Perinephric pseudocysts are formed by accumulation of transudate between the renal capsule and parenchyma in older cats as a result of underlying chronic kidney disease and can be unilateral or bilateral (**Fig. 4C**).[10,11] Sonography shows that kidneys are eccentrically located and surrounded by a large fluid-filled sac (**Fig. 9**).

Normal ureters are soft tissue opaque and 1 to 2 mm in diameter, and are not visible radiographically. They are located in the retroperitoneal space for the proximal two-thirds and peritoneal for the caudal third. If the ureter is much enlarged (hydroureter) or contains an opaque calculus (**Fig. 10**), it may be seen on a noncontrast radiograph.

Excretory Urography or Intravenous Pyelography

Nonionic organic iodides are given intravenously as a bolus and are excreted by the kidneys by glomerular filtration followed by tubular water reabsorption, which results in opacification of the diverticuli, renal pelvis, ureters, and urinary bladder (**Box 2**).[1,12] Impaired kidney function may result in increased excretion by alternate routes through the liver into bile and into the small intestine. Sequential radiographs are taken to evaluate the parenchyma and the collection system of the kidneys. Normal EU or IVP has good uniform opacification of both kidneys almost immediately (nephrogram phase; **Fig. 12A**). Very early after injection, the renal cortex may be more opaque than the renal medulla. The nephrogram phase should uniformly fade over time and be almost absent by 1 hour postinjection. The

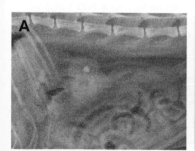
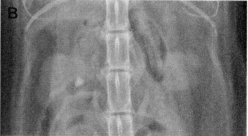

Fig. 2. (*A*) Lateral and (*B*) VD view of a cat with chronic kidney disease showing bilateral small, irregularly shaped kidneys with a well-defined renal pelvic stone in the right kidney.

Table 1
Differential diagnosis for enlarged kidneys

	Unilateral	Bilateral	Outline
Acute Kidney Injury/Pyelonephritis	—	X	Smooth
Congenital Portosystemic Shunt	—	X	Smooth
Amyloidosis	—	X	Smooth
Compensatory Hypertrophy	X	—	Smooth
Primary Neoplasia	X	—	Irregular
Metastatic Neoplasia	X	X	Irregular
Renal Lymphoma	X	X	Smooth
Perinephric Pseudocysts	X	X	Smooth
Polycystic Kidney Disease	X	X	Irregular
Renal Cysts	X	X	Irregular
Feline Infectious Peritonitis	X	X	Irregular
Hydronephrosis	X	—	—
Abscess/Hematoma	X	—	—

renal pelvis, diverticuli, and ureters should be partially visible from 5 to 45 minutes (pyelogram phase; **Fig. 12B**). Because of peristaltic activity, the entire length of the ureters is rarely visible on any 1 radiograph. EU procedures have largely been replaced by ultrasonography. However, they are the method of choice for detecting vascular, renal, or ureteral ruptures following trauma (**Fig. 13**). They are also the method of choice for depicting the ureters and in diagnosis of ectopic ureters.[4,7,9]

Ectopic ureters are congenital abnormalities of the ureteral junction with the bladder and can be unilateral or bilateral. Extramural ectopic ureters bypass the urinary bladder wall entirely and implant directly into a caudal part of the urogenital tract (**Fig. 14**). Intramural ectopic ureters are more common, tunnel caudally in the dorsal wall of the urinary bladder to the level of the urinary bladder neck or beyond, and fail to open into the lumen at the level of the trigone (**Fig. 15**).[8]

Computed tomography (CT) of the urinary tract is being used with increasing frequency in veterinary medicine and CTEU is now considered the imaging method of choice for the detection of ectopic ureters.[6–9,13,14] CT has the advantage that the entire urinary tract can be imaged accurately and noninvasively in great detail without superimposition of any other structure because of the improved spatial and temporal resolution, especially for determining the site of ureteral termination (**Fig. 15**).[7] Multiplanar and three-dimensional (3D) reconstructions add valuable information (**Fig. 16**). CT has traditionally been used in the evaluation, characterization, and surgical planning of mass effects of the abdomen and retroperitoneal space (**Fig. 17**).

Table 2
Differential diagnosis for small kidneys

	Unilateral	Bilateral	Outline
Chronic Kidney Disease	X	X	Irregular
Dysplasia/Hypoplasia	X	X	Smooth
Atrophy Secondary to Obstruction	—	X	Irregular

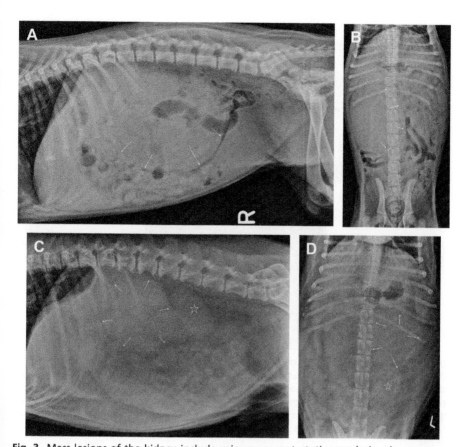

Fig. 3. Mass lesions of the kidney include primary or metastatic neoplasia, abscess, granuloma, and hematoma. Primary renal tumors include adenocarcinoma, squamous cell carcinoma, papillary carcinoma, and nephroblastoma.[29] Other tumors affecting the kidneys are histiocytic sarcoma, metastatic carcinoma, hemangiosarcoma, and lymphoma. (*A*) Lateral and (*B*) VD radiograph of a 4-month-old shepherd mix with a nephroblastoma. A well-defined, smoothly marginated, large soft tissue mass is in the right retroperitoneal space, causing the small intestines to be displaced ventral and to the left (*arrows*). (*C*) Lateral and (*D*) VD views of the abdomen of 12-year-old mixed-breed dog. Abdominal effusion is present, seen as loss of serosal detail. The left adrenal gland is enlarged (*arrows*) with a faint, linear mineralization in the periphery seen only on the VD view. The adrenal mass displaces the left kidney caudally and dorsally (*star*). An adrenal carcinoma was diagnosed.

Technique for computed tomography excretory urography

1. Sternal recumbency with slight elevation of the pelvis to pool contrast medium in urinary bladder apex away from urinary bladder neck in cases of ectopic ureters
2. Precontrast scan for evaluation of mineralization in kidney or collecting system
3. Dose 400 to 800 mg I/kg body weight of iodinated nonionic contrast agent, such as iohexol or iopromide[15]
4. Contraindication are the same as listed for EU/IVP
5. Immediate enhancement of renal parenchyma, optimal ureteral opacification occurs 3 minutes postinjection[15] and persists for about 1 hour

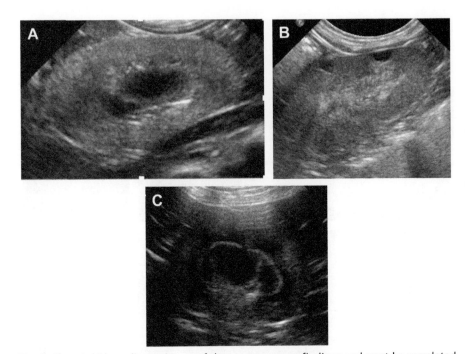

Fig. 4. Chronic kidney disease is one of the most common findings and must be correlated with clinical signs. Hyperechoic renal cortex (*A*), decreased corticomedullary definition (*B*), and small cystlike lesions (*B*) in addition to irregular margination, infarctions, and reduced size are common findings. (*C*) Hyperechoic corticomedullary rim can be seen as an incidental tubular mineralization in patients with chronic kidney disease, ethylene glycol intoxication, or with malignant hypercalcemia.

6. May have to repeat scans several times because of ureteral peristalsis for evaluation of entire ureter and ureterovesical junction

URETEROCELES

Ureteroceles are cystic dilatations of the intravesicular submucosal portion of the distal ureter. Orthotopic or intravesical ureteroceles have an orifice that communicates with the urinary bladder and they project into the lumen. Ectopic ureteroceles

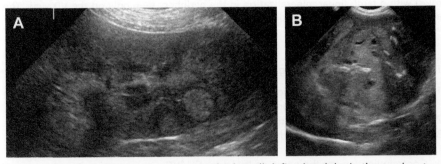

Fig. 5. (*A*) Renal neoplasia can appear as multiple well-defined nodules in the renal cortex, as seen in this longitudinal image of the left kidney of a dog with histiocytic sarcoma. (*B*) In this dog with nephroblastoma, no normal kidney architecture is appreciated.

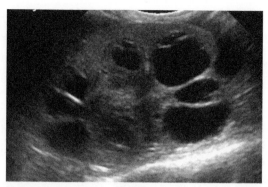

Fig. 6. Longitudinal ultrasonography image of the left kidney in a Maine coon cat. Multifocal, well-defined, thin-walled anechoic cysts with distal enhancement are present in the renal cortex consistent with polycystic kidney disease.

are associated with ectopic ureters and thus are located in an abnormal position in the urethra or urinary bladder neck.[16] In addition, a functional grading system has been proposed[16]: Grade 1 ureteroceles have no evidence of upper urinary tract disease. Grade 2 ureteroceles have ipsilateral hydroureter, hydronephrosis, or evidence of chronic kidney disease. Grade 3 ureteroceles have bilateral hydroureter, hydronephrosis, or chronic kidney disease. Grade 3 ureteroceles may arise from bilateral disease or a unilateral ureterocele that is large enough to obstruct urine outflow from the urinary bladder. Only a small number of ureteroceles have been reported in small animals.[17–21] On sonography, ureteroceles are usually smooth, round, thin-walled, cavitary, or cystic structures that contain anechoic fluid and have been described as a cyst within a cyst (**Fig. 18**).[18,19] With EU, an orthotopic ureterocele typically appears as an opacified spherical mass in the trigone region of the urinary bladder.[16,17] On positive contrast cystograms, an orthotopic ureterocele appears as a smoothly marginated filling defect in the region of the trigone.[20]

URINARY BLADDER

The canine bladder is generally pear shaped and positioned immediately cranial to the pubis on survey radiographs. The feline bladder is oval when distended; is present 2 to

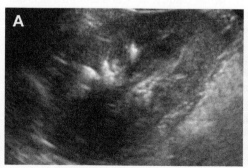
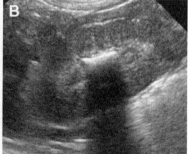

Fig. 7. Mineralization is a common finding when performing ultrasonography of the kidneys. (A) Nephrocalcinosis is noted at corticomedullary definition in this dog. (B) Nephrolithiasis is renal pelvic stone, as seen in this case with distal shadowing.

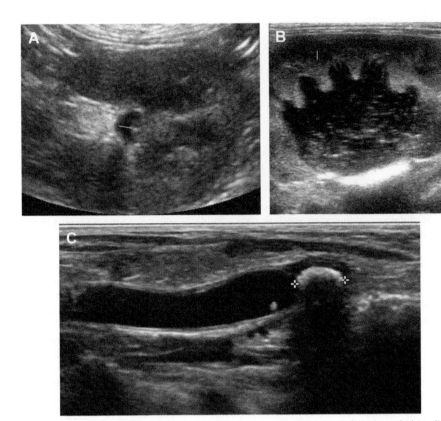

Fig. 8. (*A*) Mild renal dilatation or pyelectasia is present in this left kidney (*white line*), which is often the result of intravenous (IV) fluid administration, increased diuresis, or pyelonephritis. (*B*) Marked dilatation of the renal pelvis resulting in hydronephrosis is noted in this case. The fluid has a mixed echogenicity. Differential diagnosis includes pyelonephritis or ureteral obstruction. (*C*) Longitudinal image of the left ureter in a dog. Marked dilatation is noted to the level of ureteral stone appearing as a curvilinear, hyperechoic structure with distal shadowing (*calipers*).

3 cm cranial to the pubis; and has a long, narrow bladder neck and urethra that is outlined by fat (**Fig. 19**). On the VD view, the urinary bladder is present between the wings of the ilium and, when distended, extends into the abdomen. Urinary bladder size is extremely variable.

Sublumbar lymphadenopathy and colonic, prostatic, uterine, and bladder masses can all cause deviation in bladder position. In cases of urethral or bladder neck avulsion, the full urinary bladder is too cranially positioned and round instead of pear shaped (**Fig. 20**).

Gas in the urinary bladder is typically iatrogenic and introduced from catheterization or cystocentesis and is usually located in the center of the urinary bladder (see **Fig. 21**A). Gas in the lumen and urinary bladder wall occurs with emphysematous cystitis produced by glucose-fermenting organisms and may be seen with or without diabetes mellitus (**Fig. 21**B).[22]

Uroliths can be opaque or radiolucent and the absence of calculi on survey radiographs does not rule out their presence.[3] Calculi (**Fig. 22**) or mineralized sediment

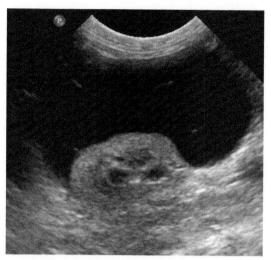

Fig. 9. Perinephric pseudocyst was diagnosed in this cat, noted by subcapsular anechoic fluid accumulation and an eccentrically located kidney with signs of chronic kidney disease with decreased corticomedullary definition.

(see **Fig. 22**D) can vary in number, size, and shape based on their composition (**Table 3**). Compression views using a wooden paddle (**Fig. 23**) or oblique views can be used to displace adjacent organs for better evaluation of the urinary bladder and suspected calculi. Ultrasonography is otherwise the imaging modality of choice in suspected urinary bladder disease processes.

Retrograde contrast cystography is a fast, simple, and inexpensive technique that may provide valuable diagnostic and prognostic information. Retrograde positive and double-contrast cystography are often more valuable to evaluate the urinary bladder than a negative retrograde cystography and the technique and indications are summarized in **Boxes 3** and **4**. Animals are best sedated or under general anesthesia. Both negative and positive contrast agents can be used for cystography (**Box 1**).

URETHRA

Survey or noncontrast radiographs of the urethra yield minimal diagnostic information except when radiopaque calculi or sediment are present (**Fig. 27**). The entire

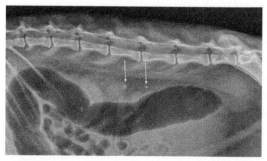

Fig. 10. Lateral radiograph of a cat presenting with ureteral obstruction. Two well-defined, round mineral opacities are noted in the ureter dorsal to colon (*arrows*).

Box 2
Excretory urogram or intravenous pyelogram

Indications for EU or IVP

- Hematuria
- Retroperitoneal mass lesion of suspected renal origin
- Ureter evaluation (ectopic or ruptured ureters)
- To evaluate urinary bladder when catheterization of bladder is impossible
- Suspected renal or ureteral trauma, retroperitoneal fluid collections

Contraindications for EU or IVP

- Patient dehydration
- Uncontrolled congestive heart failure
- Sensitivity to contrast material
- Severe kidney failure

Patient preparation

- Fast for 12 to 24 hours and cleansing enema 4 hours before study, only if elective
- Renal function within 24 hours of study, blood urea nitrogen, creatinine, urinalysis
- Assessment of hydration
- Patients should be sedated or under general anesthesia

Survey films:

- For proper positioning and radiographic technique
- Presence of too much feces (repeat enema)
- Abnormality may be present on survey films, preventing the need for contrast study
- Comparison for abnormality seen on contrast study

Contrast dose

- Bolus injection of 880 mg I per kilogram of body weight (400 mg I per pound) via indwelling catheter
- Nonionic iodinated contrast agents are safest because of lower osmolarity[30,31]

Radiographs are taken in sequence pending indication:

- Immediate VD (for arterial/venous phase)
- Five-minute VD and lateral
- Fifteen-minute VD and lateral
- Plus/minus 30-minute to 40-minute VD and lateral

Tip for ectopic ureters:

- Pneumocystogram before contrast injection and leave air in the bladder
- Elevate caudal abdomen
- Five minutes postinjection for ureterovesicular junction (**Fig. 11A, B**)
- Oblique views of the caudal abdomen

Tip for evaluation of the urinary bladder:

- Best to use 30-minute to 40-minute radiographs

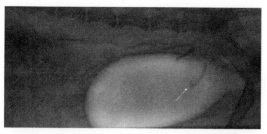

Fig. 11. Pneumocystogram with subsequent EU in this dog showing a normal ureterovesicular junction (*arrow*) entering the urinary bladder with a sharp hook.

pelvis and male urethra should be included in dogs, using 2 lateral views: one with the hind legs pulled caudally to avoid superimposition with the caudal abdomen and the other with the hind legs pulled cranially to allow full assessment of the membranous urethra without the superimposition of the stifles and muscles of the thigh (**Fig. 28**).[2,4] The urethra in females is shorter and larger in diameter than in males and a true external urethral sphincter is present. The male urethra is longer, narrower, and divided into 3 parts (**Fig. 29**): (1) the prostatic urethra extending from the urinary bladder to the caudal border of the prostate; (2) the membranous urethra from the caudal prostate gland to the caudal margin of the ischium; (3) the penile urethra from the caudal edge of the ischium to the tip of the penis. The penile urethra is smaller in diameter than the membranous urethra. The urethra runs ventral to the os penis. The penis and prepuce are located ventral to the abdominal wall in the male dog and is easily mistaken for pelvic or abdominal disorder on the VD view because it is surrounded by air and contrasts with the soft tissues (**Fig. 30**). A feline os penis is sometimes radiographically detectable in male cats and should not be mistaken for urethrolithiasis or dystrophic soft tissue mineralization (**Fig. 31**).[23]

Retrograde urethrography is the method of choice to evaluate the urethra using positive contrast medium (**Box 1**).[2,4] An overview of the technique is summarized in **Box 5**. Urethral calculi appear as focal or multifocal persistent filling defects that distend the lumen of the urethra (**Fig. 33**). Air bubbles usually are round, smoothly marginated, and not persistent on subsequent radiographs during injection (see **Fig. 33**). In cases of urethral rupture, extravasation of contrast medium in the adjacent tissues is noted (**Fig. 34**).[24,25] Strictures may occur secondary to urethral trauma (previous catheterization) or obstruction and appear as persistent luminal narrowing of the urethra (**Fig. 35**).

Ultrasonography of the urethra is usually limited to the most cranial aspect of the pelvic urethra from an abdominal approach, ideally with a distended urinary bladder, which allows evaluation of a greater length.[5] In males, the penile urethra can be imaged by using a high-frequency linear transducer (**Fig. 36**A). Cats have a longer urinary bladder neck and urethra (**Fig. 36**B). The normal urethra is smoothly marginated, thin walled, tubular, and of uniform diameter.

COMPUTED TOMOGRAPHY

As mentioned earlier, CTEU is now the method of choice in the evaluation for ectopic ureters[6–9]; however, all of the previously described urinary contrast techniques can also be performed using CT in theory and single case reports are

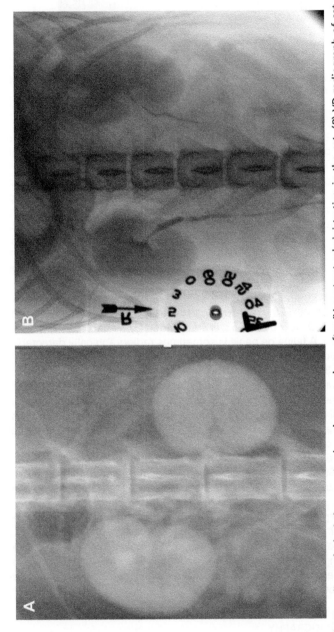

Fig. 12. (A) VD radiograph depicting a normal nephrogram phase after IV contrast administration in the cat. (B) VD radiograph of cat depicting a normal pyelogram phase with highlighted renal pelvis and ureters.

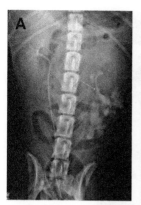
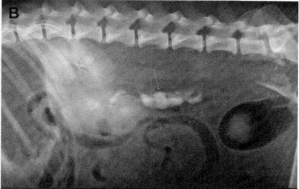

Fig. 13. (A) VD and (B) lateral views of a dog that was hit by car, resulting in multiple pelvic fractures. EU was performed and contrast leakage was noted close to the left renal pelvis (*arrow*).

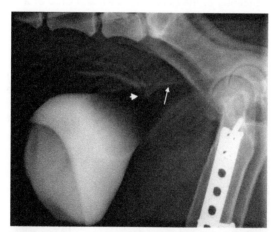

Fig. 14. Lateral radiograph of the caudal abdomen of a dog with urinary incontinence. A pneumocystogram and EU were performed. One of the ureters is noted entering the trigone (*arrowhead*) and then tunneling caudally (*arrow*), consistent with an intramural congenital ectopic ureter.

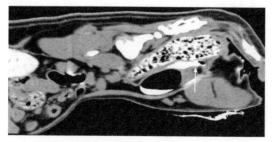

Fig. 15. CTEU was performed in this dog and a multiplanar sagittal reconstruction is shown in a soft tissue window. An extramural ectopic ureter is noted, passing past the trigone and entering the urethra in the caudal pelvis (*arrow*).

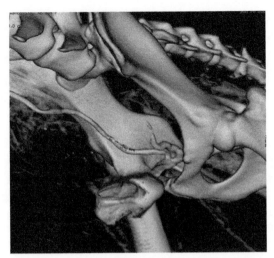

Fig. 16. 3D volume rendering of the caudal abdomen and CTEU of a dog with a complex extramural ectopic ureter inserting in the urethra.

available in veterinary medicine. CT has been described as useful in the preoperative diagnosis in 2 dogs with urinary bladder torsion, providing high anatomic detail of the point of rotation of both the pelvic urethra and urinary bladder neck, whereas ultrasonography was less helpful in these cases.[26] One other case report described the use of CT retrograde positive contrast cystography and CTEU for the diagnosis

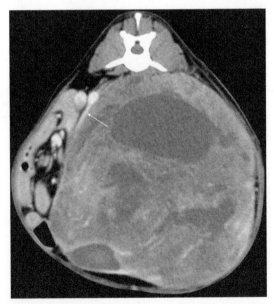

Fig. 17. Transverse postcontrast image in a soft tissue window of the abdomen in a dog with a large, complex, heterogeneous contrast-enhancing mass in the area of the left kidney. The left renal artery is seen entering the mass (*arrow*).

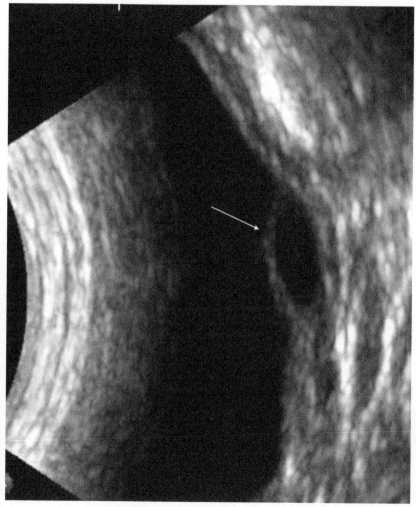

Fig. 18. Ultrasonography image of the urinary bladder in a dog with a well-defined, thin-walled, anechoic round area consistent with a ureterocele at the trigone (*arrow*) and seen as cyst within a cyst.

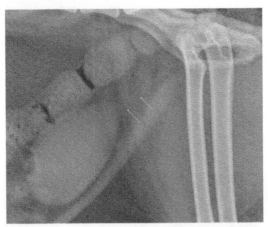

Fig. 19. Lateral radiograph of a cat with the urinary bladder neck and urethra outlined by fat (*arrows*).

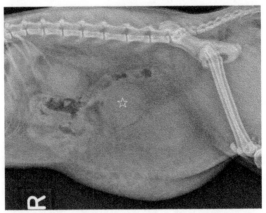

Fig. 20. Lateral radiograph of a cat that was hit by car. Increased streaky soft tissue opacity is noted in the inguinal area. The urinary bladder (*star*) is rounded and cranially displaced and the cat was diagnosed with a urethral avulsion with retrograde urethrography.

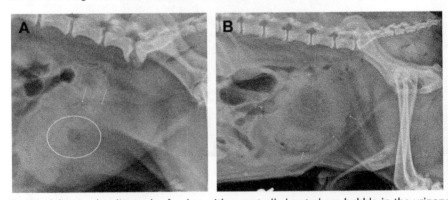

Fig. 21. (*A*) Lateral radiograph of a dog with a centrally located gas bubble in the urinary bladder from previous catheterization (*oval*). In addition, small, round mineral uroliths are present in the gravity-dependent central location of the urinary bladder (*arrows*). (*B*) Lateral radiograph of a dog with a history of recurrent urinary tract infections. Gas is outlining the wall of the urinary bladder (*arrows*) but also present in the center, consistent with an emphysematous cystitis. In addition, uroliths are present in the urinary bladder and at the base of the os penis in the urethra. The dog did not strain to urinate.

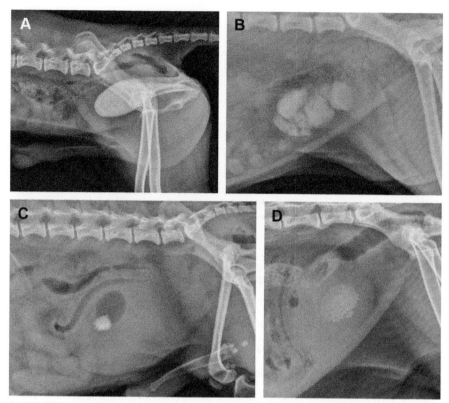

Fig. 22. (*A*) Lateral radiograph of a dog with a large, smoothly marginated stone. (*B*) Lateral radiograph in a dog with multiple variably sized uroliths. (*C*) Spiculated urolith in urinary bladder. (*D*) Multiple small mineral opaque uroliths along with sediment are present in the urinary bladder of this cat.

and preoperative characterization of a large urinary bladder diverticulum in a 1-year-old male German shepherd dog.[27] In a dog with caudal displacement of the urinary bladder with secondary trigonal invagination and urethral kinking that resulted in intermittent urethral obstruction, a combination of retrograde positive contrast cystourethrography and contrast-enhanced CT was used to characterize this complex abnormality.[28]

Table 3
Opacity of urinary bladder calculi can vary based on their composition

Composition	Opacity	Shape
Calcium oxalate	Opaque	Sharp and smooth
Calcium phosphate	Opaque	Smooth
Struvite	Opaque	Smooth, can be spiculated
Silica	Opaque	Jackstone appearance
Urate	Lucent	Smooth
Cystine	Lucent	Smooth

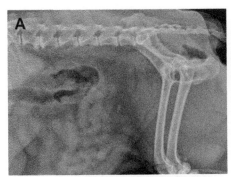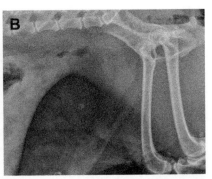

Fig. 23. (*A*) Lateral radiograph of a dog with a urolith in the urinary bladder; however, small intestines are superimposed with the apex of the urinary bladder. (*B*) A wooden spoon was used to displace the intestines and now clearly depict the stone within the urinary bladder.

Box 3
Overview of retrograde contrast cystography

1. Retrograde positive contrast cystography (**Fig. 24**A)
   Indications:
   - Suspect bladder rupture, leak, or tear
   - Locate urinary bladder, in cases of perineal hernias or abdominal wall tears
   - Abnormal communication with adjacent structures
   Technique:
   Because this is generally performed as an emergency, the patient is rarely prepared with fasting and enemas.
   - Survey radiographs of the caudal abdomen are obtained and evaluated
   - Catheterize and evacuate urinary bladder
   - Iodinated contrast medium solution (20%) is injected into the bladder (assess by palpation)
   - Lateral and oblique VD views are obtained during injections
   - If the bladder is not intact, the contrast medium will be seen in the peritoneal space (**Fig. 24**B)

2. Retrograde double-contrast cystography
   Indications:
   - Suspect radiolucent cystic calculi
   - Suspect bladder tumor or polyps
   - Suspect chronic cystitis
   - Suspect urachal diverticuli
   Contraindications:
   Because of the possibility of fatal air embolization, this procedure should not be performed in patients with severe bladder hemorrhage.
   Technique:
   This is rarely an emergent procedure, so patient preparation is important.
   - Survey radiographs
   - Catheterize and completely empty the urinary bladder
   - Fill the bladder with carbon dioxide or room air until the bladder is distended (assess by palpation)
   - Instill 4 to 12 mL of iodinated contrast medium into the bladder; 36% iodine solutions work best
   - Roll animal gently to coat the bladder mucosa with contrast
   A normal double-contrast cystogram shows an oval radiolucent urinary bladder with a radiopaque, smooth inner mucosal surface and a radiopaque, central, gravity-dependent contrast puddle (**Fig. 25**).[3,4,32]

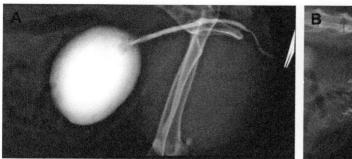
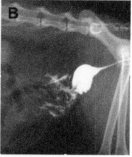

Fig. 24. (*A*) Normal positive cystourethrogram in a cat. (*B*) Retrograde positive cystography in a cat showing extravasation of contrast at the apex.

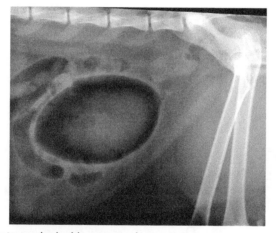

Fig. 25. Normal retrograde double cystography.

Box 4
Retrograde negative contrast cystography or pneumocystogram (Fig. 26)

Indications:
- Suspect ectopic ureters, the study is done in conjunction with EU or IVP
- Suspect bladder mass

Contraindications:
  Because of the possibility of fatal air embolization, this procedure should not be performed in patients with severe bladder hemorrhage or in cases of suspected bladder rupture.

Technique:
- Catheterize urinary bladder and drain
- Inflate bladder with 30 to 300 mL, depending on the size of patient, until moderately distended (assess by palpation)
- Lateral and oblique VD views are obtained after injection

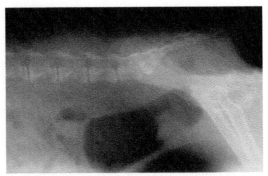

Fig. 26. Retrograde negative cystogram in a dog with a urinary bladder tumor visible at the level of the urinary bladder neck.

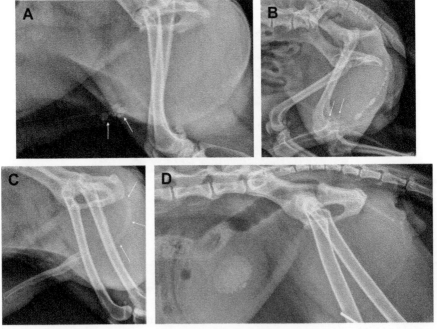

Fig. 27. (A) Multiple, variably sized and shaped mineral calculi (*arrows*) are present in this dog at the base of the os penis. Calculi commonly occur at regions of luminal narrowing: ischial arch and the base of the os penis, as seen in this dog. (B) In this dog, multiple urethral calculi are present from the ischial arch to the os penis. Note the superimposition of the fabellae (*arrows*) caused by obliquity of the radiograph. (C) In this survey radiograph in a dog, faint mineralized sediment is seen in the penile urethra (*arrows*). (D) Lateral survey radiograph of a male cat with obstruction. Note the multiple small mineral calculi in the urinary bladder and urethra, outlining the position of the feline male urethra to show the importance of including the entire pelvis and perineal area in the view.

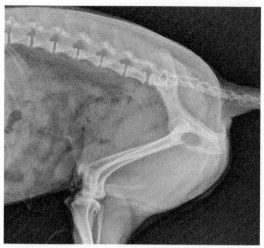

Fig. 28. Lateral radiograph of a male dog with the hind legs pulled cranial to eliminate superimposition of the thighs with the urethra.

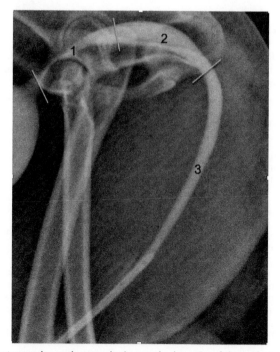

Fig. 29. Normal retrograde urethrography in a male dog. Tip of the catheter is at the base of the os penis. The urethra is divided into the (1) the prostatic urethra; (2) The membranous urethra; (3) and the penile urethra.

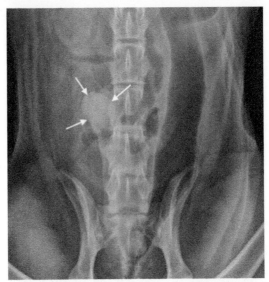

Fig. 30. The prepuce is outlined by gas and seen as well-defined soft tissue opacity on VD views (*arrows*) and often mistaken for an abdominal lesion.

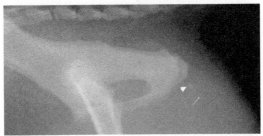

Fig. 31. Lateral radiograph of an obstructed male cat. Well-defined round mineral opacity is present in the urethra (*arrowhead*) in addition to faint linear mineral opacity that could represent additional urethral calculi or an os penis (*arrow*).

Box 5
Retrograde urethrography

Indications:
- Dysuria, stranguria, hematuria.
- Suspect urethral rupture or calculi (nonradiopaque).
- Suspect urethral obstruction, urethritis, or urethral tumor.

Technique:
- Cleansing enema 4 hours before performing this procedure.
- Sedation of the patient is advised for easier and faster image acquisition.
- The most distal urethra is catheterized with a Foley or balloon-tipped urethral catheter.[24,25] Carefully inflate to a pressure that will not damage the urethra and leave inflated no more than 15 minutes.[33]
- Fully distended urinary bladder provides counterpressure to contrast medium injection to allow for maximal distention of the urethra.[34]
- Often cystography is performed first, and distention of the urinary bladder should be maintained. Sterile saline can be used to maximize distention of an inadequately filled urinary bladder.
- Dilute 15% or 150 mg I/mL iodinated contrast medium is injected as a moderately forceful bolus.[24]
- Depending on patient size, a total of 5 to 20 mL of contrast medium needed.
- Lateral and oblique VD films are taken during injection. It is imperative to make the radiograph exposure while actively injecting so the urethra is distended (**Fig. 32**).

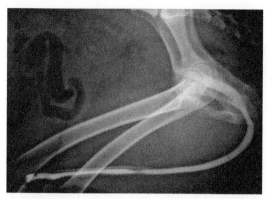

Fig. 32. Normal retrograde urethrogram in a male dog, showing a smooth-walled tube of radiopaque contrast of similar diameter.

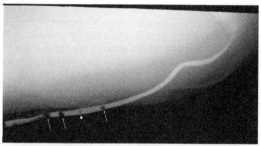

Fig. 33. Retrograde urethrography in a dog with nonradiopaque uroliths. The catheter is seen at the tip of the os penis. Multifocal, slightly irregular filling defects are present that distend the urethra (*arrows*) representing uroliths, as well as 1 well-defined round gas bubble (*arrowhead*) that was in a different position on subsequent images (not shown).

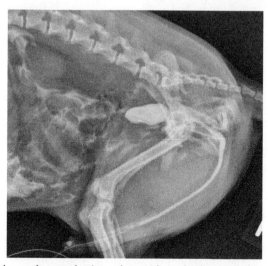

Fig. 34. Retrograde urethrography in a dog with multiple pelvic fractures caused by a vehicle accident. The catheter was placed at the level of the os penis and contrast was injected. At the level of the membranous urethra, and the pelvic floor fractures, extravasation of contrast into the abdominal cavity outlining small intestinal loops of bowel as well as the perineal area is present.

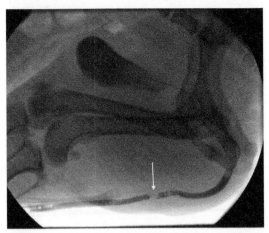

Fig. 35. Fluoroscopic retrograde urethrogram in a dog straining to urinate. Persistent narrowing of the lumen of the penile urethra is present proximal to the os penis (*arrow*) with multiple gas bubbles that disappeared on subsequent injections. A diagnosis of urethral stricture was made.

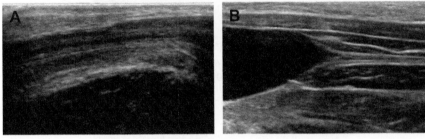

Fig. 36. (*A*) Longitudinal ultrasonography image of the normal penile urethra in a male dog using a linear transducer. (*B*) Longitudinal ultrasonography image of the urinary bladder neck and urethra in a normal cat, showing the long neck and smoothly marginated urethra.

SUMMARY

Survey radiographs are still being used as a screening method because of the ease of the modality. Ultrasonography is the main modality of choice for an initial work-up, followed by contrast radiology, whereas now CTEU is the modality of choice for evaluation for ectopic ureters.

REFERENCES

1. Seiler GS. Kidneys and ureters. In: Thrall D, editor. Textbook of veterinary diagnostic radiology. 7th edition. St. Louis, Missouri: Elsevier; 2018. p. 823–45.
2. Brown J. Urethra. In: Thrall D, editor. Textbook of veterinary diagnostic radiology. 7th edition. St. Louis, Missouri: Elsevier; 2018. p. 865–70.
3. Marolf A. Urinary bladder. In: Thrall D, editor. Textbook of veterinary diagnostic radiology. 7th edition. St. Louis, Missouri: Elsevier; 2018. p. 846–64.
4. Baines E. Practical contrast radiography 3. Urogenital studies. In Pract 2005;27: 466–73.

5. Nyland T, Widmer W, Mattoon J. Urinary tract. In: Matton J, Nyland T, editors. Small animal diagnostic ultrasound. 3rd edition. St Louis (MO): Elsevier; 2015. p. 557–607.
6. Anders KJ, McLoughlin MA, Samii VF, et al. Ectopic ureters in male dogs: review of 16 clinical cases (1999-2007). J Am Anim Hosp Assoc 2012;48(6):390–8.
7. Samii VF, McLoughlin MA, Matton J, et al. Digital fluoroscopic excretory urography, digital fluoroscopic urethrography, helical computed tomography, and cystoscopy in 24 dogs with suspected ureteral ectopia. J Vet Intern Med 2004; 18:271–81.
8. Fox AJ, Sharma A, Secrest SA. Computed tomographic excretory urography features of intramural ectopic ureters in 10 dogs. J Small Anim Pract 2016;57(4): 210–3.
9. Rozear L, Tidwell AS. Evaluation of the ureter and ureterovesicular junction using helical computed tomographic excretory urography in healthy dogs. Vet Radiol Ultrasound 2003;44(2):155–64.
10. Ochoa VB, DiBartola SP, Chew DJ, et al. Perinephric pseudocysts in the cat: a retrospective study and review of the literature. J Vet Intern Med 1999;13(1): 47–55.
11. Beck JA, Bellenger CR, Lamb WA, et al. Perirenal pseudocysts in 26 cats. Aust Vet J 2000;78(3):166–71.
12. Kneller S. Role of the excretory urogram in the diagnosis of renal and ureteral disease. Vet Clin North Am Small Anim Pract 1974;4(4):843–61.
13. Longo M, Andreis ME, Pettinato C, et al. Use of the bolus tracking technique for the tomographic evaluation of the uretero-vesicular junction in dogs and assessment of dose records. BMC Vet Res 2016;12:64.
14. Seiler GS. The kidneys and ureters. In: Thrall D, editor. Textbook of veterinary diagnostic radiology. 6th edition. St. Louis, Missouri: Saunders; 2013. p. 705–25.
15. Barthez PY, Begon D, Delisle F. Effect of contrast medium dose and image acquisition timing on ureteral opacification in the normal dog as assessed by computed tomography. Vet Radiol Ultrasound 1998;39(6):524–7.
16. Stiffler KS, Stevenson MAM, Mahaffey MB, et al. Intravesical ureterocele with concurrent renal dysfunction in a dog: a case report and proposed classification system. J Am Anim Hosp Assoc 2002;38(1):33–9.
17. Tattersall JA, Welsh E. Ectopic ureterocele in a male dog: a case report and review of surgical management. J Am Anim Hosp Assoc 2006;42(5):395–400.
18. Takiguchi M, Yasuda J, Ochiai K, et al. Ultrasonographic appearance of orthotopic ureterocele in a dog. Vet Radiol Ultrasound 1997;38(5):398–9.
19. Secrest S, Britt L, Cook C. Imaging diagnosis-bilateral orthotopic ureteroceles in a dog. Vet Radiol Ultrasound 2011;52(4):448–50.
20. McLoughlin MA, Hauptman J, Spaulding KA. Canine ureteroceles: a case report and literature review. J Am Anim Hosp Assoc 1989;25:699–706.
21. Hoffman S, Ferguson H, Flanders J. Bilateral ectopic ureters in a male dog: a case report. J Am Anim Hosp Assoc 1985;21:80–4.
22. Root CR, Scott RC. Emphysematous cystitis and other radiographic manifestations of diabetes mellitus in dogs and cats. J Am Vet Med Assoc 1971;158(6): 721–8.
23. Piola V, Posch B, Aghte P, et al. Radiographic characterization of the os penis in the cat. Vet Radiol Ultrasound 2011;52(3):270–2.
24. Ticer J, Spencer C, Ackerman N. Positive contrast retrograde urethrography: a useful procedure for evaluation urethral disorders in the dog. Vet Radiol Ultrasound 1980;21(1):2–11.

25. Pugh CR, Rhodes WH, Biery DN. Contrast studies of the urogenital system. Vet Clin North Am Small Anim Pract 1993;23(2):281–306.
26. Ricciardi M, Campanella A, Martino R. Computed tomographic features of urinary bladder torsion in two dogs. J Small Anim Pract 2018;59(3):188–95.
27. Anson A, Strohmayer C, Larrinaga JM, et al. Computed tomographic retrograde positive contrast cystography and computed tomographic excretory urography characterization of a urinary bladder diverticulum in a dog. Vet Radiol Ultrasound 2018. https://doi.org/10.1111/vru.12591.
28. Kanakubo K, Palm C, Korner A, et al. Treatment of urethral obstruction secondary to caudal bladder displacement, trigonal invagination, and urethral kinking in a dog. J Am Vet Med Assoc 2017;251:818–23.
29. Bryan JN, Henry CJ, Turnquist SE, et al. Primary renal neoplasia of dogs. J Vet Intern Med 2006;20(5):1155–60.
30. Pollard RE, Puchalski SM, Pascoe PJ. Hemodynamic and serum biochemical alterations associated with intravenous administration of three types of contrast media in anesthetized cats. Am J Vet Res 2008;69(10):1274–8.
31. Pollard RE, Puchalski SM, Pascoe PJ. Hemodynamic and serum biochemical alterations associated with intravenous administration of three types of contrast media in anesthetized dogs. Am J Vet Res 2008;69(10):1268–73.
32. Johnston GR, Feeney D. Comparative organ imaging: lower urinary tract. Vet Radiol Ultrasound 1984;25(4):146–53.
33. Johnston GR, Stevens JB, Jessen CR, et al. Complications of retrograde contrast urethrography in dogs and cats. Am J Vet Res 1983;44(7):1248–56.
34. Johnston GR, Jessen C, Osborne C. Effects of bladder distention on canine and feline retrograde urethrography. Vet Radiol Ultrasound 1983;24(6):271–7.

Interventional Therapies of the Urinary Tract

Emmanuelle Butty, DMV[a], Catherine Vachon, DMV, DVSc[b], Marilyn Dunn, DMV, MVSc[c],*

KEYWORDS

- Interventional endoscopy • Interventional radiology • Endourology • Fluoroscopy
- Image-guided interventions

KEY POINTS

- Minimally invasive interventional therapies are the new standard of care in veterinary medicine.
- In comparison with standard surgical procedures, they are associated with minimal tissue injury, leading to shorter, smoother recovery and decreasing the perioperative morbidity and mortality.
- A thorough understanding of the therapeutic options available is essential to properly educate and inform clients.
- Proper equipment, technical expertise, and experience are essential prerequisites to many of these procedures.

 Video content accompanies this article at http://www.vetsmall.theclinics.com.

INTRODUCTION

Minimally invasive procedures for the treatment of congenital, acquired, and neoplastic conditions of the urinary tract began to emerge 20 years ago and have become increasingly available in veterinary medicine. Interventional urology, or endourology, refers to the specialty of urology in which endoscopes, fluoroscopy, and other instruments are used to access, under direct visualization, structures inside the urinary tract. Access is most commonly achieved through natural orifices and the procedures are done internally either without or with minimal external incisions. Minimally invasive approaches have a multitude of advantages over standard surgery, such as shorter hospitalization times, little to no recovery time, and less discomfort.

Disclosure: The authors have nothing to disclose.
[a] Cummings School of Veterinary Medicine, Tufts University, 200 Westboro Rd, North Grafton, MA 01536, USA; [b] Centre Hospitalier Universitaire Vétérinaire, University of Montreal, Saint-Hyacinthe, Quebec, Canada; [c] Centre Hospitalier Universitaire Vétérinaire, Faculty of Veterinary Medicine, University of Montreal, 1525 Rue des Vétérinaires, Saint-Hyacinthe, QC J2S 8H5, Canada
* Corresponding author.
E-mail address: marilyn.dunn@umontreal.ca

Vet Clin Small Anim 49 (2019) 287–309
https://doi.org/10.1016/j.cvsm.2018.10.002
0195-5616/19/© 2018 Elsevier Inc. All rights reserved.

The authors believe that minimally invasive procedures should be considered, discussed, and offered to owners of pets suffering from urinary tract conditions (**Fig. 1**). Although at times appearing technically simple, these procedures have been associated with serious complications when performed by inadequately trained personnel and should be referred to a formally trained and experienced specialist.

This article reviews the current minimally invasive treatment options for management of some lower urinary tract conditions (urolithiasis, urinary incontinence, urethral obstructions, and bladder masses). The purpose of this article is to introduce the reader to veterinary interventional urology. Please consult the references for detailed procedural and technical information.[1]

Urolithiasis of the upper urinary tract are discussed in Melissa Milligan and Allyson C. Berent's article, "Medical and Interventional Management of Upper Urinary Tract Uroliths," in this issue.

The procedures described should be performed in a sterile manner. Patients should be clipped and aseptically prepared and all instruments entering the urinary bladder should be sterile.

LOWER URINARY TRACT UROLITHIASIS

Removal of lower urinary tract urolithiasis is amenable to various interventional approaches depending on the species, gender, type of stone present, and stone burden. Consideration of minimally invasive approaches to stone removal in lieu of surgical cystotomy is recomended[2] (**Fig. 2**).

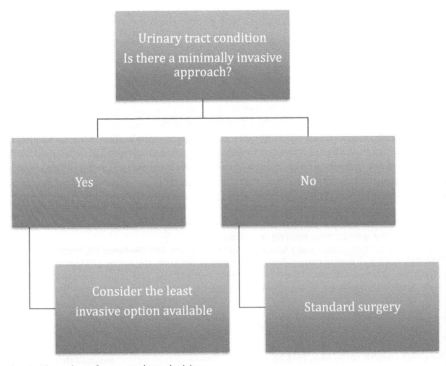

Fig. 1. Flow chart for procedure decisions.

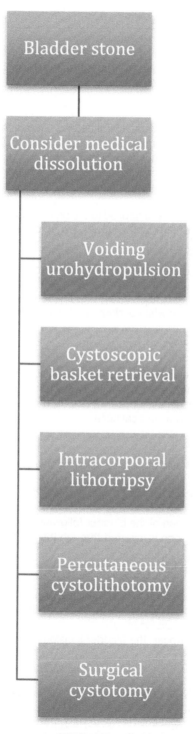

Fig. 2. Algorithm for the recommended approach to lower urinary tract urolithiasis removal.

Voiding Urohydropulsion

Indications

This procedure should be considered for antegrade removal of bladder stones through the urethra. This procedure is recommended for small stones in female cats and dogs but should not be attempted in male cats[3] (**Table 1**).

Intervention

- Under general anesthesia, a urinary catheter is used to fill the bladder with saline (avoid overfilling; estimated bladder capacity 10–15 mL/kg).
- The urinary catheter is removed; in female cats and dogs, the patient is positioned vertically whereas male dogs are placed in lateral recumbency.
- The urinary bladder is palpated, shaken gently, and pulled cranially to straighten the urethra.
- Gentle but steady pressure is applied to the urinary bladder to induce micturition.
- Repeat the procedure until all the stones are removed.

Complications

This procedure is generally well tolerated, however, mild hematuria may be noted. Careful urinary bladder palpation while filling with saline is recommended to prevent overfilling and bladder rupture. Inadvertent urethral obstruction due to numerous uroliths being voided may occur while performing the procedure.

Percutaneous Cystolithotomy

Indications

This procedure is indicated for urolith removal of any size/number in dogs and cats of any breed, gender, and size. Percutaneous cystolithotomy can be considered when uroliths are too large to be removed by urohydropulsion[4] (see **Table 1**). This procedure must be done aseptically in a surgical suite.

Intervention

- Under general anesthesia, a urinary catheter is placed and the bladder is filled with saline.
- An abdominal incision, 1 cm to 1.5 cm, is made over the bladder apex.
- The bladder apex is exposed, stay sutures are placed, and a screw trocar is advanced into the lumen of the bladder following a stab incision at the apex.
- Rigid/flexible cystoscope is inserted through the trocar under continuous saline irrigation.
- A stone basket passed through the working channel of the cystoscope is used to remove the stones.
- Lithotripsy may be needed to fragment large or embedded stones.
- In male cats and dogs, all or most of the urethra can be examined in an antegrade manner with a flexible cystoscope.
- After removal of the trocar, the bladder incision is closed in a standard manner (**Fig. 3**).

Other considerations

Laser lithotripsy is rarely required because larger cystoliths may be removed by stretching/extending the bladder incision. This procedure can be performed on an outpatient basis. If a patient has a urinary tract infection, antibiotic therapy should be administered prior to the procedure due to increased risk of septic peritonitis.

Table 1
Summary of minimally invasive options for the removal of lower urinary tract urolithiasis in cats and dogs

	Size and Number of Uroliths	Gender and Species	Advantages	Disadvantages
Voiding urohydropulsion	Stones <3–4 mm in small female dogs Stones <2.5 mm in female cats Male dogs limited by size of penile urethra	Female dogs and cats Not indicated in male cats	Quick Low cost equipment	Stones may remain in the bladder Large and spiculated stones may obstruct the urethra
PCCL	No restrictions	No restrictions	Excellent visualization of the entire lower urinary tract and easy retrograde stone removal	Specialized equipment Access to lithotripsy may be necessary for large or embedded stones
Cystoscopic basket retrieval	Stones <4–5 mm in small female dogs Stones <3 mm female cats Male dogs limited by size of penile urethra (2–3 mm)	Female dogs and cats Male dogs >7 kg (penile urethra must allow passage of the flexible scope)	Quick No suture material in the bladder	Specialized equipment
Intracorporal lithotripsy	Low stone burden preferable	Female cats and dogs Male dogs >7 kg	No suture material in the bladder	Specialized equipment Long procedural length with large stone burden

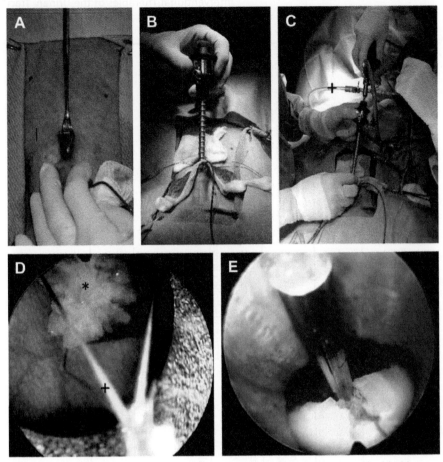

Fig. 3. Various steps in a PCCL in a male dog. A 1.5-cm incision is made over the bladder apex in a male dog with a urinary catheter (*A*). A trocar is inserted into the apex of the bladder following a stab incision (*B*). A rigid cystoscope (*asterisk*) is inserted through the trocar under continuous saline irrigation (*plus*) (*C*). A stone basket retrieval device (*plus*) passed through the working channel of the endoscope allows stone (*asterisk*) retrieval from the bladder (*D*). A lithotripsy probe passed through the working channel of the endoscope fragments an embedded urethral stone (*E*).

Complications

Urine leakage due to inadequate bladder wall closure is rare but may occur. Careful cystoscopic evaluation of the urethra and bladder minimizes the risk of incomplete stone removal (3.7% in 1 study).[4]

Cystoscopy and Intracorporal Lithotripsy

Indications

This procedure is indicated for urolith removal in female dogs and cats and some male dogs (see **Table 1**).

Male cats, small male dogs, and patients with large stone burdens should undergo percutaneous cystolithotomy (PCCL).

Intervention

- Under general anesthesia, a retrograde urethrocystoscopy is performed.
- Smaller uroliths are removed using a stone basket.

- Larger uroliths are fragmented by a holmium:YAG laser or electrohydraulic lithotripter (Video 1). Direct contact of the tip of the laser fiber is required. Once fragments are small enough, they can be removed using the stone retrieval basket. Smaller fragments and debris can also be voided by urohydropulsion.[5,6]

Complications

Cystoscopy and intracorporal lithotripsy in a patient with a urinary tract infection is not recommended due to increased risk of urosepsis. Antibiotic therapy based on culture/ sensitivity is recommended for 5 days to 7 days prior to performing this procedure.

Potential complications include urethral tears, strictures, and bleeding. Bladder wall damage and perforation are possible complications but can be limited by avoiding contact of the laser/lithotripter with the urethral or bladder mucosa. Risk of incomplete stone fragment removal is higher in male cats and dogs (20%–30%) than in female cats and dogs due to the difficulty in removing stone fragments by voiding urohydropulsion in male dogs.[5,6]

URINARY INCONTINENCE
Cystoscopic Guided Laser Ablation of Intramural Ectopic Ureters

Ectopic ureters (EUs) are characterized by 1 or both ureters inserting at a site outside of the bladder. Intramural EUs enter the bladder wall normally but tunnel distally in the submucosa through the trigone before inserting caudal to the urethral sphincter. Extramural EUs bypass the bladder before ending caudal to the urethral sphincter. The recorded locations of ectopia in dogs are the vesicourethral junction, proximal portion of the urethra, midurethra, distal portion of the urethra, and vestibule, with a majority (45.8%) identified in the distal urethra.[7] In male dogs, the vesicourethral junction, preprostatic, and prostatic urethra have been recorded with a majority (36%) identified in the preprostatic urethra.[8]

Indications

Because greater than 95% of EUs are intramural in female dogs, cystoscopic guided transurethral laser ablation (CLA) of intramural EU has emerged as a minimally invasive alternative to surgical correction and become the standard of care. Male dogs may have a higher incidence of extramural ectopia and, therefore, a retrograde cystourethrogram is essential to confirm the intramural course of the ureter prior to laser ablation.[9,10] This procedure must be done aseptically in a surgical suite.

Intervention

- Cystoscopy, vaginoscopy, and fluoroscopy-guided retrograde cysto-urethroureterograms are performed under anesthesia to identify the site of the ectopia, identify concurrent anomalies, and confirm the intramural course of the EU (**Fig. 4**).
- A laser fiber, holmium:YAG, or diode, is inserted through the operating channel of the cystoscope.
- The medial wall of the EU is transected until the ureteral orifice inserts cranial to the urethral sphincter well within the trigone (**Fig. 5**).
- If a vestibulovaginal remnant is present, laser ablation of the remnant can be done during the same procedure (**Fig. 6**).
- Correction of EU in male dogs can be technically challenging and often requires a percutaneous perineal approach.

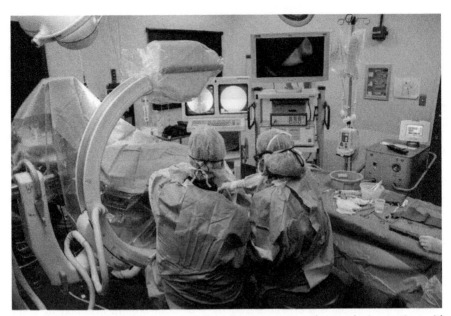

Fig. 4. Fluoroscopic guided assistance while performing cystourethrography in a patient with EU. Note the integrated approach of using fluoroscopy and cystoscopy during the procedure.

Other considerations

Diagnosis is made/confirmed by cystoscopy and fluoroscopic guided retrograde ureterogram. Advanced imaging, such as CT, is rarely required unless other anomalies are suspected (vascular).[11,12]

Treatment of lower urinary tract infections is recommended prior to CLA.[11] Dogs with EU frequently have various other anomalies of the genitourinary tract (eg, vestibulovaginal remnants [93%], urethral sphincter mechanism incompetence [USMI], hypoplastic bladder, and pelvic bladder). Incontinence may persist after the procedure because of these concurrent urinary tract anomalies.[11,12]

Complications

Perforation of the lower urinary tract is a rare occurrence and can be treated by leaving a urinary catheter in place for 24 hours to 48 hours. After the procedure, patients can present with self-limiting mild dysuria and pollakiuria; 30% of dogs are diagnosed with a urinary tract infection within 6 months after the procedure.[11]

Outcome

CLA results in continence rates of 47% in female dogs 6 months after the procedure. Continence rates increase to 77% with the addition of medical, cystoscopic, or surgical therapy for USMI.[11] Success rates are higher in male dogs (83%–100%).[8,12] The procedure is well tolerated and can be done on an outpatient basis. CLA has similar treatment outcomes compared with open surgical management and recurrence of the ectopia and stricture at the site of the new ureterovesicular orifice, the main complication with surgical management, has been rarely reported with CLA.

PERCUTANEOUS PERINEAL ACCESS
Indications

The percutaneous perineal access procedure is performed in male dogs greater than 10 kg (urethra must accommodate a 14F–16F peel-away sheath) allowing rigid

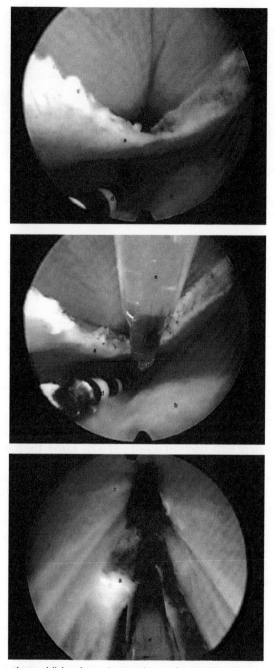

Fig. 5. A ureteral catheter (d) has been inserted into the EU (*Top Panel*), the medial wall of the EU (a) is excised with a diode laser (e) (*Middle Panel*). The lateral wall of the EU, which is also the lateral wall of the urethra, is visible (b). The bladder lumen is visible (c) (*Bottom Panel*).

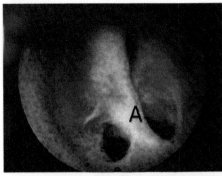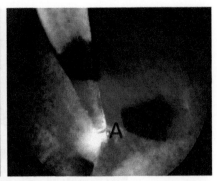

Fig. 6. Cystoscopic view of a female dog placed in dorsal recumbency undergoing cystoscopy with a vestibulovaginal remnant (A) (*Left Panel*). A holmium:YAG laser is ablating the remnant (*Right Panel*).

urethrocystoscopy of the prostatic urethra and bladder. Rigid scope access to these structures facilitates ureteral stenting, treatment of renal hematuria, ureteroscopy, injection of urethral bulking agents, and so forth. This procedure must be done aseptically in a surgical suite.

Intervention

- Patient is placed in dorsal recumbency with the hindlimbs pulled cranially.
- Urethroscopy is performed using flexible endoscopy to ensure normal urethral anatomy.
- A 4-mm to 5-mm midline skin incision is performed at the level of the pelvic urethra and ischium. A combination of ultrasound or digital transrectal palpation and fluoroscopic assistance is used to help guide the procedure.
- A Foley catheter (8F) is advanced in the bladder and pulled back toward the ischial urethra. The bladder and urethra are filled with saline and contrast
- Using a mixture of 50% contrast agent and 50% saline, the balloon of the Foley catheter is filled to occlude the urethral lumen.
- An 18-gauge renal puncture needle is aimed at puncturing the balloon of the Foley catheter (transrectal palpation of the urethra/balloon may help stabilize the balloon to facilitate puncture).
- Once the urethral lumen is accessed, a guide wire is advanced in the urinary bladder and serial dilations are performed until the peel-away sheath (14F or 16F) is placed (**Fig. 7**).
- At the end of the procedure, the peel-away sheath is removed and the perineal incision heals by second intention.

Complications

Complications may occur, including mild hemorrhage at the puncture site. Urethral strictures have not been reported. In 1 study involving 19 dogs, excellent outcomes and no complications were noted in 84% of dogs; 16% reported urine leakage at the site of perineal access for 48 hours. Other minor complications included irritation at the site of perineal access and stranguria for a couple of days.[13]

Urethral Sphincter Mechanism Incompetence

USMI is the most common cause of incontinence in adult dogs (particularly in female dogs, after ovariohysterectomy) and is second only to ureteral ectopia in young

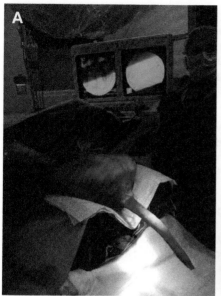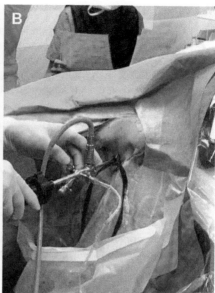

Fig. 7. A male dog is placed in dorsal recumbency with the hind legs pulled forward, a Foley catheter has been placed in the bladder/urethra, and the perineal region has been aseptically prepared (*A*). A peel-away urethral access sheath is placed in the perineal urethra allowing passage of a rigid cystoscope under continuous saline flush (*B*).

dogs.[14] Although urethral pressure profilometry has to be performed to demonstrate incompetence of the urethral sphincter mechanism,[15] this technique is not readily available in general practice and the diagnosis is typically made through a process of elimination and response to therapy.

Medical therapy

Medical treatment of USMI includes an α-agonist, estrogens, or both. Phenylpropanolamine (PPA) is an α_1-agonist that improves urethral tone via its sympathomimetic effect. Diethylstilbestrol and estriol are synthetic estrogens that improve urethral tone by sensitizing the urethral sphincter to α_1-adrenoreceptors (see Mark J Acierno and Mary Anna Labato's article "Canine Incontinence," in this issue).

Although response rates for PPA and estrogen are reported to be up to 97% and 93%, respectively, these treatments are not without reported side effects.[16,17] Interventional therapies are available for treatment of refractory cases or when side effects occur.

Urethral Bulking Agents

Submucosal injection of bulking agents in the proximal urethra improves continence by acting as an additional central filler, which increases the length of the muscle fiber and thereby the strength of the sphincter.[18] The major drawbacks of urethral bulking agents are lack of sustained efficacy and, therefore, the need for repeated injections.

Indication

The injection of urethral bulking agents is mainly indicated in older female dogs with USMI refractory to medical therapy, given the ease and minimal invasiveness of the technique.

Intervention

- The procedure is performed under general anesthesia via cystoscopy.
- The urethral bulking agent (collagen or Teflon-based products have been used in veterinary medicine) is injected submucosally in 3 to 5 locations until blebs result in occlusion of the urethral lumen (**Fig. 8**) (please see Mark J Acierno and Mary Anna Labato's article, "Canine Incontinence," in this issue).

Complications

The injection of urethral bulking agents is well tolerated; however, incontinence may persist. Inability to urinate is infrequent and if occurs, can be treated with placement of an indwelling urethral catheter for 24 hours to 48 hours. Acute allergic reaction has rarely been reported with polydimethylsiloxane.[19]

Prognosis

A major disadvantage of urethral bulking agents is the poor long-term response with a mean duration of 17 months to 21 months.[20–22] Continence rates using collagen in female dogs vary from approximately 60% to 75% when treated concurrently with an α-agonist. If patients remain incontinent, a second injection of a bulking agent can be performed.

Artificial Urethral Sphincter

Indications

Placement is indicated in dogs and cats with USMI refractory to medical therapy.

Intervention

The artificial urethral sphincter (AUS) is placed surgically around the urethra and connected to an access port placed subcutaneously on the ventral body wall (**Fig. 9**).

Other considerations

The cuff is first left empty because approximately 30% to 45% of dogs may be continent after placement of the AUS device alone due to passively increased urethral tone from the implant.[23,24] If incontinence persists 4 weeks to 6 weeks postoperatively, saline is injected into the subcutaneous access port using a Huber needle to inflate the silicone cuff until continence is improved or signs of urethral obstruction occur. Cystoscopy and urinary catheter placement should be avoided perioperatively and postoperatively because it may induce mucosal lesions, increasing the chance of intraluminal stricture formation.

Complications

Minor complications include temporary worsening of incontinence during the first 14 days after surgery (19%), mild stranguria (7%), and seroma formation over the access port (11%). Urinary tract infections are observed in 61% of female dogs during long-term follow-up. Urinary obstruction is a major complication requiring AUS removal and has been reported 1.5 months to 23 months postoperatively.[23,24] Two dogs required urethral stenting to treat extraluminal urethral strictures in 1 study.[23]

Prognosis

AUS results in high continence rates in dogs[23–25] (90%) and a long-term response.[25] AUS have been placed successfully in both female and male dogs and cats.[26]

URETHRAL OBSTRUCTION

Diagnosis of urethral obstruction is commonly based on presentation and physical examination findings; however, to confirm obstruction and identify its site and cause

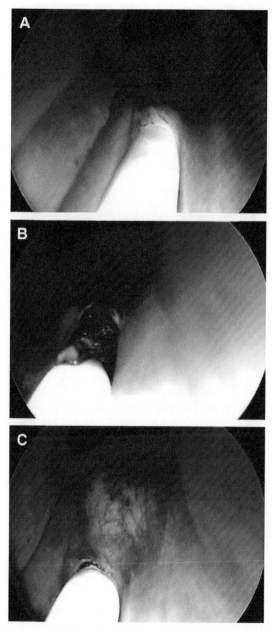

Fig. 8. Cystoscopic assisted injection of a bulking agent in the proximal urethra of a female dog diagnosed with USMI. An injection needle is passed through the working channel of the cystoscope, the needle tip is inserted into the mucosa (*A*). Injection of the bulking agent creates a bleb thus decreasing the size of the urethral lumen, a small amount of the bulking agent can be seen leaking around the injection needle (*B*). Injection of the bulking agent is continued until a bleb is seen and there is blanching of the mucosa (*C*).

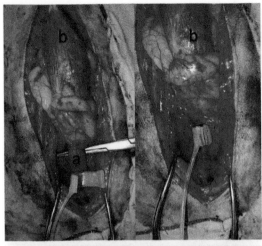

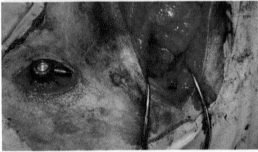

Fig. 9. Surgical placement of an AUS. The urethra is identified (a) measured and the proper size occluder is placed around the urethra and closed with a suture passing through the eyelets (*Top Panel*). The tubing is passed through the abdominal wall and connected to the port sutured to the ventral rectus sheath (*Bottom Panel*).

requires imaging (ultrasound, contrast radiography, cystoscopy, CT, or MRI). This section discusses cystourethrography, urethral stenting, tumor ablation, and placement of a cystostomy tube.

Cystourethrography

Indications

The cystourethrography procedure is performed to investigate the cause of urethral obstruction and voiding phase abnormalities in cats and dogs. It is commonly performed to investigate urethral stricture, tear, spasms, radiolucent urethral stones, lower urinary tract neoplasia (intraluminal or extraluminal neoplasia), and reflex dyssynergia (**Figs. 10** and **11**).

Intervention

- Patient is placed in lateral recumbency and aseptically prepared.
- A marker catheter is placed within a red rubber urinary catheter, placed in the colon to allow for measurements.
- A guide wire is advanced in the urethra and curled into the urinary bladder under cystoscopic/fluoroscopic guidance.
- A urethral or vascular sheath (most commonly 8F) should be used.

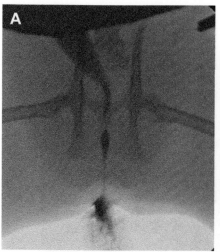
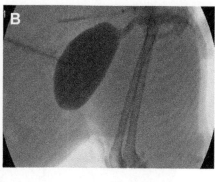

Fig. 10. Voiding cystourethrogram in a male cat with a midurethral stricture (*A*). Cystoureth-rogram in a male cat with a distal penile urethral stricture. The cat could not be catheter-ized; therefore, bladder filling was accomplished by injecting contrast through a 22-gauge catheter directly into the bladder (*B*).

- In male dogs, the Berenstein catheter is advanced in the urethra through the sheath to inject the contrast agent.
- In female dogs, the contrast agent is administered directly through the sheath.
- Using a mixture of 50:50 iodinated contrast agent and sterile saline 0.9%, a contrast cystourethrogram is performed.
- Full urinary bladder filling is required to delineate the bladder trigone and prox-imal urethra.
- Once the bladder is distended, the contrast agent is continuously injected while the Berenstein catheter is withdrawn under fluoroscopic guidance.
- Manual bladder compression may help in performing a proper voiding cystour-ethrogram because it maximizes urethral distension.

Other considerations
In patients with suspected reflex dyssynergia/urethral spasms, however, sedation may aid in localizing the site(s) of obstruction. If retrograde catheterization is not possible, an antegrade approach through the bladder with fluoroscopic guidance has been described.[26,27]

Complications
Complications are uncommonly encountered with cystourethrography. Bladder rupture/leakage due to over distension or improper handling is rare. Inadequate bladder distention with contrast and the lack of a voiding phase result in a poorly filled urethra, which could be misinterpreted as a stricture or spasm.[1]

Urethral Stenting

Indications
Urethral stenting is performed in patients with partial/complete urinary obstruction due to urethral, trigonal, or prostatic (or combination of) neoplasia.[28–31] Patients with ure-thral stricture or proliferative urethritis may require stenting especially if they have

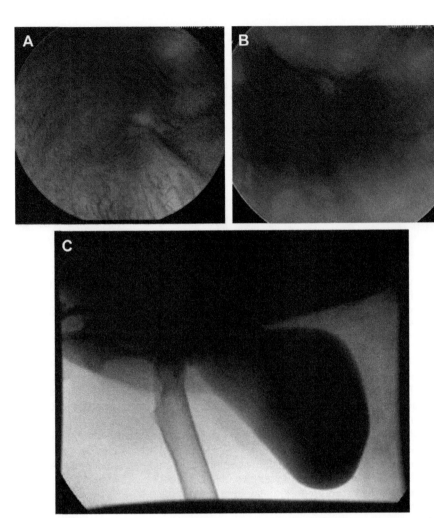

Fig. 11. Urethral stricture in a female dog seen on cystoscopy (*A*). Cystoscopic image of the urethral stricture post–balloon dilatation (*B*). Cystourethrogram of the same dog showing a proximal urethral stricture prior to balloon dilatation (*C*).

failed ballooning and medical therapy.[28,32,33] Rarely, patients with refractory urethral spasms/reflex dyssynergia may benefit from urethral stenting[28,32] (**Figs. 12** and **13**).

Intervention

- Urethral stenting is performed under general anesthesia and fluoroscopic guidance.
- A radio-opaque measuring catheter is placed in the colon in order to calculate the measurements required for urethral stenting.
- Measurements of the length of the obstruction and width of the unaffected portion of the urethra are used to select stent size.
- The stent is passed over a guide wire, into position, and deployed under fluoroscopic guidance to relieve the obstruction.

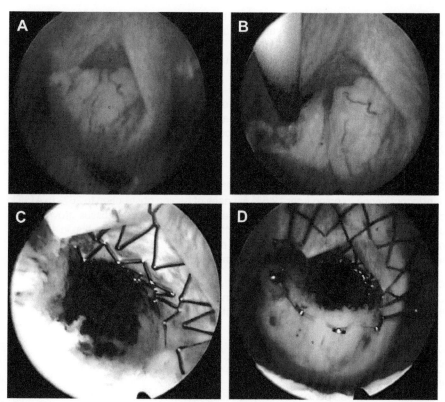

Fig. 12. Obstructive soft tissue mass invading the distal urethra and papilla in a female dog (a, vagina; b, urethral lumen; and c, soft tissue mass at the urethral papilla) (*A*). A guide wire is passed into the urethral lumen to gain access to the urethra and bladder (*B*). A urethral stent is in place restoring patency to the urethral lumen. The soft tissue mass is pushed open by the stent (*C*). The stent is seen protruding from the urethral papilla (*D*).

Other considerations

For benign urethral obstruction, balloon dilatation may be considered prior to urethral stenting. For recurrent benign urethral obstruction, a covered stent may be required to prevent tissue ingrowth.

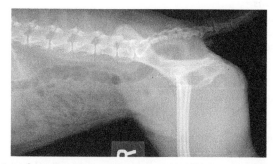

Fig. 13. Same patient from **Fig. 12**. A urethral stent is visible spanning the distal two-thirds of the urethra.

In patients with trigonal neoplasia resulting in both urethral and ureteral obstructions, subcutaneous ureteral bypass or ureteral stenting may be required at the time of urethral stent placement. Extensive trigonal/urethral neoplasia can also be addressed by excision of the bladder, urethra and ureters and placement of a neobladder.

Metallic urethral stents are considered permanent implants. Removable urethral stents can be used to maintain urethral patency in patients with treatable or temporary conditions (proliferative urethritis). A permanent cystotomy or temporary pigtail catheter sutured to the vestibule or prepuce are other means of relieving urethral obstruction.

Complications
The most common complications include urinary tract infection in a third of cases and urinary incontinence, ranging from 12.5% in cases of benign obstruction to 26% to 41% in cases of malignant obstruction. Recurrence of obstruction due to tissue growth (more common with benign strictures) occurs in 12.8% to 17%, stent migration in 12%, and persistent dysuria and stranguria in 19% of patients.[28–33] Given the location of their ureteral orifices, a proximal urethral stent placement in cats can lead to ureteral obstruction.[34]

Outcome
Urethral stenting is a safe and successful method to relieve benign and malignant urethral obstruction, with a success rate greater than 95%.[29,31,32]

URETHRAL/BLADDER MASSES
Laser Ablation

Indications
Laser ablation can be performed for debulking/removal of both neoplastic and benign bladder and urethral masses. Ablation may reestablish a urine stream in cases of complete malignant obstruction (**Fig. 14**).

Intervention
- Laser ablation is performed under general anesthesia and ultrasound guidance.
- Cystoscope is advanced to within 2 mm to 5 mm of the tumor to allow precise viewing and control of the laser fiber.
- Ultrasonographic monitoring to allow tumor ablation without penetration of the bladder or urethral wall (masses in the distal two-thirds of the urethra are not visible on ultrasound).

Other considerations
The resulting denatured, avascular tissue sloughs within several days. Either a diode or holmium:YAG laser can be used for ablation. The user should be familiar with various contact and noncontact modes to facilitate ablation while providing hemostasis.

Complications
Perforation of the bladder or urethral wall can lead to tumor seeding of the abdomen and require hospitalization with a urinary catheter.

Prognosis
Long-term success with laser ablation of bladder and urethral polyps has been reported.

Ablation of transitional cell carcinomas has been described and is referred to as ultrasound-guided endoscopic laser ablation (UGELAB).[35] This procedure is

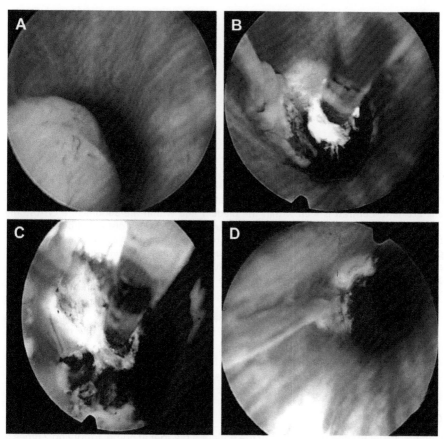

Fig. 14. A single urethral mass diagnosed as transitional cell carcinoma is seen on cystoscopy partially obstructing the urethral lumen (*A*). A diode laser is used to ablate the mass. Progressive steps in mass ablation (*B, C*). Cystoscopic view of the urethra after ablation of the mass (*D*).

considered palliative, and chemotherapy should be maintained to improve outcome (mean survival time of 380 days).[35] Despite relief of urethral obstruction, many dogs remain persistently dysuric and pollakiuric, which can improve over time. Bacterial cystitis (reported in 50% of cases postoperatively) or tumor regrowth/spread should be considered if lower urinary tract signs recur. Patients may undergo multiple laser treatments and follow-up ultrasound can aid in early identification of tumor recurrence.

PERCUTANEOUS CYSTOSTOMY TUBES
Indications

A cystostomy tube can be used as a temporary or permanent implant to drain the bladder in patients with urethral, trigonal, and prostatic neoplasia; granulomatous urethritis; urethral stricture; dyssynergia; neurologic disease; and urethral/bladder trauma.[36,37] They can also serve as a temporary option allowing bladder emptying while the underlying disorder is corrected (**Fig. 15**).

Intervention

- Cystostomy tubes can be placed surgically or percutaneously with fluoroscopic guidance. Locking loop pigtail catheters are most commonly used.

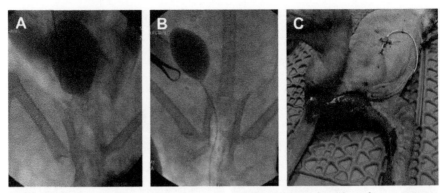

Fig. 15. Placement of a cystostomy tube in a cat with a transected urethra after an automobile accident. Contrast is seen within the bladder and within the abdomen, a cystostomy tube placed over a guide wire is inserted percutaneously into the distended bladder under fluoroscopic-guidance (*A*). The loop of the cystostomy tube is visible and the guide wire is passed through the urethra resulting in through and through access (*B*). The cystostomy tube is seen exiting the abdominal wall and sutured in place. Sloughing of the perineum occurred secondary to urine scalding from the ruptured urethra (*C*).

- The bladder is accessed with a needle and filled with contrast; a guide wire is looped in the bladder and passed through the urethra until through-and-through access is achieved.
- The needle is withdrawn and the locking loop catheter is passed over the guide wire.
- The guide wire is removed allowing the loop to be formed and the string locked. The tube should be left in place 10-14 days before removing.

Other Considerations

Owners are instructed how to empty the patient's bladder at home. Emptying 2 times a day to 3 times a day is recommended.

Complications

Patients with cystostomy tubes have a high rate of bacterial urinary tract infections (86%), especially when undergoing chemotherapy for malignant obstructions.[37] Bacterial urinary tract infections should only be treated when associated with clinical signs and with targeted antimicrobial therapy based on culture and sensitivity. Other common complications include inadvertent tube removal, ingestion of the tube by the patient, fistula formation, and catheter breakage.[38]

Prognosis

The authors have successfully managed permanent cystotomy tubes in patients in place for years.

PERCUTANEOUS ANTEGRADE URETHRAL CATHETERIZATION
Indications

Percutaneous antegrade urethral catheterization is indicated when a urethral obstruction cannot be relieved by standard retrograde catheterization or when animals are difficult or too small to catheterize or have a urethral tear or a distal urethral obstruction. It is most commonly performed in male cats with iatrogenic urethral tears secondary to trauma from serial attempts to catheterize. Because the tear is made in a longitudinal retrograde direction, the antegrade passage is effective.

Intervention

- General anesthesia and fluoroscopic guidance
- Intravenous catheter percutaneously inserted into the apex of the full urinary bladder.
- Passage of a guide wire in an antegrade manner through the catheter, the bladder then down the urethra until it exits through the penis or vulva
- Catheter withdrawn from the bladder apex.
- Urinary catheter advanced in a retrograde manner over the guide wire until it reaches the bladder.
- Guide wire is removed.

Other Considerations

In cases of urethral tears, the urinary catheter should be left in place for 1 to 10 days (the authors recommend 3–5 days based on personal experience) to allow complete healing.[27]

Complications

The main complication is the inability to achieve access and urine leakage into the abdomen if the obstruction is not relieved.

Prognosis

A small study on percutaneous antegrade urethral catheterization in male cats was successful in 7 of 9 cats, but all of these cats underwent perineal urethrostomy for recurrence of urethral obstruction within 6 weeks.[27]

SUMMARY

Minimally invasive interventional therapies are the new standard of care in veterinary medicine. In comparison with standard surgical procedures, they are associated with minimal tissue injury, leading to shorter, smoother recovery and decreasing the perioperative morbidity and mortality. A thorough understanding of the therapeutic options available is essential to properly educate and inform the client. Proper equipment, technical expertise, and experience are essential prerequisites to many of these procedures. For detailed procedural descriptions, please refer to the book edited by Weisse and Berent[1] and the chapter by Dunn and Berent[26] and contact a veterinary interventionalist.

SUPPLEMENTARY DATA

Supplementary data related to this article can be found online at https://doi.org/10.1016/j.cvsm.2018.10.002.

REFERENCES

1. Weisse C, Berent A. Veterinary image-guided interventions. Wiley-Blackwell; 2015.
2. Lulich JP, Berent AC, Adams JL, et al. ACVIM small animal concensus recommendations on the treatment and prevention of uroliths in dogs and cats. J Vet Intern Med 2016;30:1564–74.

3. Lulich JP, Osborne CA, Carlson M. Nonsurgical removal of uroliths in dogs and cats by voiding urohydropropulsion. J Am Vet Med Assoc 1993;203:660–3.

4. Runge JJ, Berent AC, Mayhew PD, et al. Transvesicular percutaneous cystolithotomy for the retrieval of cystic and urethral calculi in dogs and cats: 27 cases (2006-2008). J Am Vet Med Assoc 2011;239:344–9.

5. Adams LG, Berent AC, Moore GE, et al. Use of laser lithotripsy for fragmentation of uroliths in dogs: 73 cases (2005-2006). J Am Vet Med Assoc 2008;232:1680–7.

6. Defarges A, Dunn M. Use of electrohydraulic lithotripsy to treat bladder and urethral calculi in 28 dogs. J Vet Intern Med 2008;22:1267–73.

7. Cannizzo KL, McLoughlin MA, Mattoon JS, et al. Evaluation of transurethral cystoscopy and excretory urography for diagnosis of ectopic ureters in female dogs: 25 cases (1992-2000). J Am Vet Med Assoc 2003;223(4):475–81.

8. Anders KJ, McLoughlin MA, Samii VF, et al. Ectopic ureters in male dogs: review of 16 clinical cases (1999–2007). J Am Anim Hosp Assoc 2012;48(6):390–8.

9. Holt PE, Moore AH. Canine ureteral ectopia: an analysis of 175 cases and comparison of surgical treatments. Vet Rec 1995;136(14):345–9.

10. Burdick S, Berent A, Weisse C, et al. Endoscopic-guided laser ablation of vestibulovaginal septal remnants in Dogs: 36 cases (2007-2011). J Am Vet Med Assoc 2014;244(8):944–9.

11. Berent AC, Weisse C, Mayhew PD, et al. Evaluation of cystoscopic-guided laser ablation of intramural ectopic ureters in female dogs. J Am Vet Med Assoc 2012; 240(6):716–25.

12. Berent AC, Mayhew PD, Porat-Mosenco Y. Use of cystoscopic-guided laser ablation for treatment of intramural ureteral ectopia in male dogs: four cases (2006-2007). J Am Vet Med Assoc 2008;232(7):1026–34.

13. Tong K, Weisse C, Berent AC. Rigid urethrocystoscopy via a percutaneous fluoroscopic-assisted perineal approach in male dogs: 19 cases (2005-2014). J Am Vet Med Assoc 2016;249:918–25.

14. Holt PE. Urinary incontinence in dogs and cats. Vet Rec 1990;127(14):347–50.

15. Holt PE. Simultaneous urethral pressure profilometry: comparisons between continent and incontinent bitches. J Small Anim Pract 1988;29(12):761–9.

16. Blendinger C, Blendinger K, Bostedt H. Urinary incontinence in castrated female dogs. 2. Therapy. Tierarztl Prax 1995;23(4):402–6 [in German].

17. Janszen BPM, van Lear PH, Bergman JGHE. Treatment of urinary incontinence in the bitch: a pilot field study with incurin®. Vet Q 1997;19(1):42.

18. Klarskov N, Lose G. Urethral injection therapy: what is the mechanism of action? Neurourol Urodyn 2008;27(8):789–92.

19. Bartges JW, Callens A. Polydimethylsiloxane urethral bulking agent (PDMS UBA) injection for treatment of female canine urinary incontinence - preliminary results. J Vet Intern Med 2011;2:492.

20. Barth A, Reichler IM, Hubler M, et al. Evaluation of long-term effects of endoscopic injection of collagen into the urethral submucosa for treatment of urethral sphincter incompetence in female dogs: 40 cases (1993-2000). J Am Vet Med Assoc 2005;226(1):73–6.

21. Byron JK, Chew DJ, Mcloughlin ML. Retrospective evaluation of urethral bovine cross-linked collagen implantation for treatment of urinary incontinence in female dogs. J Vet Intern Med 2011;25(5):980–4.

22. Arnold S, Hubler M, Lott-Stolz G, et al. Treatment of urinary incontinence in bitches by endoscopic injection of glutaraldehyde cross-linked collagen. J Small Anim Pract 1996;37(4):163–8.

23. Currao RL, Berent AC, Weisse C, et al. Use of a percutaneously controlled ure-thral hydraulic occluder for treatment of refractory urinary incontinence in 18 fe-male dogs. Vet Surg 2013;42(4):440–7.

24. Reeves L, Adin C, Mcloughlin M, et al. Outcome after placement of an artificial urethral sphincter in 27 dogs. Vet Surg 2013;42(1):12–8.

25. Rose SA, Adin CA, Ellison GW, et al. Long-term efficacy of a percutaneously adjustable hydraulic urethral sphincter for treatment of urinary incontinence in four dogs. Vet Surg 2009;38(6):747–53.

26. Dunn M, Berent A. Chapter 124 interventional urologic therapies in textbook of veterinary internal medicine. 8th edition. Philadelphia, PA: Saunders Elsevier; 2016. p. 493–512.

27. Holmes ES, Weisse C, Berent AC. Use of fluoroscopically guided percutaneous antegrade urethral catheterization for the treatment of urethral obstruction in male cats: 9 cases (2000-2009). J Am Vet Med Assoc 2012;241(5):603–7.

28. Radhakrishnan A. Urethral stenting for obstructive uropathy utilizing digital radi-ography for guidance: feasibility and clinical outcome in 26 dogs. J Vet Intern Med 2017;31:427–33.

29. Blackburn AL, Berent AC, Weisse CW, et al. Evaluation of outcome following ure-thral stent placement for the treatment of obstructive carcinoma of the urethra in dogs: 42 cases (2004-2008). J Am Vet Med Assoc 2013;242:59–68.

30. Weisse C, Berent A, Todd K, et al. Evaluation of palliative stenting for manage-ment of malignant urethral obstructions in dogs. J Am Vet Med Assoc 2006; 229:226–34.

31. McMillan SK, Knapp DW, Ramos-Vara JA, et al. Outcome of urethral stent place-ment for management of urethral obstruction secondary to transitional cell carci-noma in dogs: 19 cases (2007–2010). J Am Vet Med Assoc 2012;241:1627–32.

32. Hill TL, Berent and AC, Weisse CW. Evaluation of urethral stent placement for benign urethral obstructions in dogs. J Vet Intern Med 2014;28:1384–90.

33. Della Maggiore AM, Steffey MA, Westropp JL. Treatment of traumatic penile ure-thral stricture in a dog with a self-expanding, covered nitinol stent. J Am Vet Med Assoc 2013;242:1117–21.

34. Brace MA, Weisse C, Berent A. Preliminary experience with stenting for manage-ment of non-urolith urethral obstruction in eight cats. Vet Surg 2014;43(2): 199–208.

35. Cerf DJ, Lindquist EC. Palliative ultrasound-guided endoscopic diode laser abla-tion of transitional cell carcinomas of the lower urinary tract in dogs. J Am Vet Med Assoc 2012;240(1):51–60.

36. Salinardi BJ, Marks SL, Davidson JR, et al. The use of a low-profile cystostomy tube to relieve urethral obstruction in a dog. J Am Anim Hosp Assoc 2003; 39(4):403–5.

37. Smith JD, Stone E a, Gilson SD. Placement of a permanent cystostomy catheter to relieve urine outflow obstruction in dogs with transitional cell carcinoma. J Am Vet Med Assoc 1995;206(4):496–9.

38. Beck AL, Grierson JM, Ogden DM, et al. Outcome of and complications associ-ated with tube cystostomy in dogs and cats: 76 cases (1995-2006). J Am Vet Med Assoc 2007;230(8):1184–9.

Urologic Oncology

Kristine Elaine Burgess, DVM[a],*, Carol J. DeRegis, DVM, PhD[b]

KEYWORDS

- Renal • Bladder • Neoplasia • Carcinoma • Transitional cell carcinoma

KEY POINTS

- Primary renal tumors are uncommon in small animals, and as a consequence only a few retrospective studies describing biologic behavior and metastatic potential exist.
- Treatment of primary renal cancers include surgery ± adjuvant chemotherapy. Prognosis is directly dependent on tumor type and presence of metastatic disease.
- Transitional call carcinoma (TCC), a primary bladder or urethral neoplasia, is more prevalent and can serve as a strong comparative model for humans with invasive bladder cancer.
- Presenting clinical signs are similar to that described for primary renal tumors but treatment centers on adjuvant chemotherapy and COX-2 inhibitors.
- Interventional surgery, such as stenting and laser ablation, is used in a palliative setting to address tumor-associated urinary obstruction.

PRIMARY RENAL TUMORS

Urologic neoplasia including primary renal tumors and tumors of the bladder or urethra are uncommon in domestic animals accounting for less than 1% of all neoplastic conditions and 2% of malignant tumors.[1–3]

Primary renal tumors are especially rare, estimated to be only 0.3% of all canine neoplasms, with secondary or metastatic neoplasia from other locations having a more frequent occurrence.[1–3] Renal cell carcinoma (RCC), arising from the epithelial cells of the nephron, is the most common primary kidney tumor in dogs, accounting for 49% to 65% of primary renal tumors. Other tumor types include various sarcomas or on rare instances, nephroblastoma.[1–4]

A review of the literature suggests prognosis is directly dependent on tumor subtype and therapy pursued. As expected, dogs that present with widespread metastases at the time of diagnosis have shorter survival times as compared with dogs with no

---

Disclosure Statement: The authors have nothing to disclose.
[a] Department of Clinical Science, Cummings School of Veterinary Medicine, Tufts University, 200 Westboro Road, North Grafton, MA 01536, USA; [b] Piper Memorial Veterinary Center, 730 Randolph Road, Middletown, CT 06457, USA
* Corresponding author.
E-mail address: Kristine.burgess@tufts.edu

evidence of metastasis with an extended survival of up to 4 years following nephrectomy.[1–8]

Renal Cell Carcinoma

Because of the relative infrequency of this diagnosis, only a few retrospective studies describing biologic behavior and metastatic potential of RCC exist.[3,4] Presenting clinical signs may be nonspecific and include lethargy, anorexia, polyuria/polydipsia, abdominal pain, or cachexia. In advanced cases, a palpable abdominal mass may be detected on routine physical examination. Overall, hematuria is the most common presenting sign occurring in 32% of patients. Azotemia is the most frequent biochemical alteration developing late in the course of the disease; other blood parameter alterations are uncommon. There are isolated reports of dogs presenting with polycythemia syndrome as a paraneoplastic condition secondary to RCC.[3]

Overall, RCC, as with most primary renal cancers, can be a clinically silent disease (eg, the primary tumor can reach a considerable size before clinical signs are apparent), consequently it is often diagnosed late in the course of disease.[3,4] It has a moderate metastatic rate (16%–34%) at the time of diagnosis and a higher metastatic rate (70%–75%) in the late stage of disease. Metastatic sites include the contralateral kidney, abdominal organs, omentum/peritoneum, and lungs. Approximately 5% of patients present with bilateral kidney involvement.[1–4]

To better understand the biologic behavior of renal carcinoma, a histologic evaluation was conducted on the kidneys of 70 dogs after nephrectomy.[4] The authors classified carcinomas into four subtypes based on histologic features and histochemical and immunohistochemical staining: (1) clear cell, (2) chromophobe, (3) papillary, and (4) multilocular cystic RCC. Clear cell carcinoma, accounting for 9% of cases, was associated with a significantly decreased survival time (median, 87 days).[4] This study demonstrated that mitotic index (MI), defined as the number of mitotic figures in 10 fields ×400, was the sole independent prognostic variable. In this study, the median survival time for dogs with an MI greater than 30 was 187 days compared with 1184 days for dogs with an MI of less than 10, whereas dogs with an intermediate MI (10–30) had a median survival time of 452 days.

Nephroblastoma

A tumor of embryonic tissue, nephroblastoma, has been reported in young dogs (<2 year old) as either a primary renal tumor or as a tumor within the thoracolumbar portion of the spinal cord.[1,6,7] This tumor has been described in humans and is often referred to as Wilms tumor.[6–8] The tumor arises from neoplastic transformation during nephrogenesis or from nephrogenic nests that persist postnatally.[1–3,6–8] As with other kidney tumors there is a paucity of information in the literature with one small case series of five dogs with primary renal nephroblastoma, which reported a median survival time of 6 months; however, scattered case reports document long-term survival with surgery ± chemotherapy.[8]

Renal Cystadenocarcinomas

A unique syndrome has been described in German shepherd dogs consisting of bilateral, multifocal renal cystadenocarcinomas and nodular dermatofibrosis.[1–3] Affected dogs present with multiple subcutaneous fibrous nodules, uterine leiomyomas, and multiple renal adenocarcinomas/adenomas.[1–3] This disorder seems to have an autosomal-dominant mode of inheritance associated with a gene localized to chromosome 53 believed to be a mutation in the folliculin gene.[9] A similar condition has been described in people and is referred to as Birt-Hogg-Dube syndrome. This disease process is characterized by multiple noncancerous skin tumors and is believed to be associated with a mutation in the folliculin gene.[9]

Renal Sarcomas

An older study evaluating primary renal tumors in dogs included a group of 28 dogs with multiple subtypes of renal sarcomas including hemangiosarcoma (12), renal sarcoma (seven), leiomyosarcoma (four), malignant fibrous histiocytoma (three), spindle cell sarcoma (one), and fibroleiomyosarcoma (one).[3] All dogs in this study were treated with nephrectomy ± chemotherapy and had a median survival time of 9 months, compared with 16 months for those with carcinomas, although this difference did not reach statistical significance. The metastatic rate was 14% at diagnosis and 88% at the time of death for this population of dogs.[3]

Primary renal hemangiosarcoma has also been described in the veterinary literature.[10] Similar to other organs affected with hemangiosarcoma, dogs in this study were treated with surgical removal of the tumor followed by chemotherapy.[10] However, the efficacy of adjuvant chemotherapy for this tumor type has not yet been established.

Treatment of Primary Renal Tumors

Regardless of tumor type, successful management of primary renal neoplasia centers on complete excision of the mass.[1,3–10] Because of the high metastatic risk, some form of adjuvant chemotherapy is typically recommended. Specific protocols recommended are dependent on exact tumor type, and for most there is no standard of care, thus treatment is often empiric and based on clinician experience and studies from the human literature.

Because of the poor response rates to conventional chemotherapy in human patients with RCC, this tumor type may have inherent resistance to conventional cytotoxic agents.[5] Nevertheless survival times have improved considerably with the use of novel therapeutic agents, such as small molecular inhibitors, antiangiogenic drugs, and immunotherapies in humans with RCC.[5] Currently, interleukin-2 and interferon serve as the mainstay of treatment of this disease in humans.[5] Data are lacking to support the use of these therapies in canine patients but anecdotal experience suggests the small molecule inhibitor toceranib phosphate may have some efficacy in controlling this disease process.

There is one study of 14 dogs with renal hemangiosarcoma that reported a median survival time of approximately 9 months with a 1-year survival rate of 29% for dogs treated with surgical excision ± a doxorubicin-based chemotherapy treatment protocol.[10] This study demonstrated a significantly shorter median survival time (62 days vs 286 days) for dogs presenting with a hemoabdomen versus those who did not.[10]

Nephroblastoma has been anecdotally treated with various adjuvant therapies, but because of the rarity of this tumor in veterinary medicine, there is not yet a protocol that has been defined as superior to others.

RENAL LYMPHOMA

Renal lymphoma is an uncommon diagnosis in cats. It usually causes bilateral renomegaly, which may be detected on physical examination. Clinical signs at presentation are a consequence of renal insufficiency.[1,11] Ultrasound-guided renal biopsy or fine-needle aspiration is recommended to confirm the diagnosis.

Treatment consists of a standard multiagent chemotherapy protocol. However, because many cats with renal lymphoma have or will develop central nervous system involvement, treatment with a multiagent protocol incorporating a drug with central nervous system penetration (eg, CCNU) is recommended.

TUMORS OF THE URINARY BLADDER AND URETHRA

Tumors of the bladder and urethra account for approximately 0.5% to 1.0% of all canine neoplasms. Approximately 90% of bladder tumors are malignant and 75% to 90% of primary urinary bladder epithelial tumors are transitional cell carcinomas (TCC). Other possible tumor types include squamous cell carcinoma, adenocarcinoma, rhabdomyosarcoma, leiomyoma, or leiomyosarcoma.[1–3,12]

TRANSITIONAL CELL CARCINOMA

TCC typically arises from the trigone of the bladder, urethra, or prostate. Most commonly these tumors are solitary, although they can be invasive and cover a large portion of the bladder mucosa.[1–3,12–17]

Incidence and Risk Factors

Female dogs are reported to outnumber males by approximately 2:1 and neutered animals of either gender have approximately four times the risk of their intact counterparts.[1,2,12–15] Certain breeds of dogs are considered at high risk for developing TCC, including Scottish Terriers, West Highland White Terriers, Shetland sheepdogs, beagles, and other terrier breeds.[1,2,12–15]

Pesticide exposures are a recognized environmental risk factor for TCC in dogs.[18–21] Diet and body condition have also been evaluated as risk factors for the development of TCC with overweight animals having three times increased risk compared with lean dogs.[20,22] Notably, the consumption of vegetables in Scottish terriers was found to decrease the risk to about one-third that for those not regularly consuming vegetables.[22]

Although the chemotherapy drug cyclophosphamide and environmental tobacco exposures are established risk factors for TCC in humans, a cause and effect relationship has not been established in dogs; however, TCC has been reported in three dogs with prior exposure to cyclophosphamide.[23]

Clinical Signs and Physical Examination Findings

TCC in dogs has a predilection for the bladder trigone resulting in lower urinary tract signs indistinguishable from those observed with urolithiasis or lower urinary tract infection and may include stranguria, hematuria, pollakiruia, and tenesmus.[1–3,12–15] As a result, TCC is often diagnosed late in the disease process because many dogs can have a transient response to empiric antibiotic therapy or anti-inflammatory medications.

Physical examination abnormalities may include a distended bladder; a mass or thickening of the bladder, urethra, or vagina; prostatomegaly; or internal lymph node enlargement. A digital rectal examination is critical in the assessment of TCC because a portion of the urethra is shielded from routine imaging techniques, such as ultrasound.

Diagnostic Tests

Noninvasive diagnostics include a urinalysis, urine culture, urine cytology, bladder tumor antigen evaluation, and testing for the presence of a BRAF mutation.[24–27] It is highly recommended that cystocentesis be avoided in all at-risk breeds of dogs or dogs with a known bladder mass because of the risk of needle track implantation.[28,29]

Relying solely on an evaluation of a voided urine sample to establish a definitive diagnosis is not recommended because reactive hyperplastic transitional cells can have a pleomorphic appearance indistinguishable from that of malignant cells.

The commercially available bladder tumor antigen test can support a diagnosis of TCC, although false-positive results are obtained when there is significant proteinuria, glucosuria, pyuria, or hematuria.[24–26] Given the potential for false-positive results, this test is often used to screen at-risk populations with a 93% negative predictive value and 27% positive predictive value in this setting.[24,25]

A new diagnostic test that relies on the molecular detection of a genetic alteration is now available. This test, which is completed on a voided urine sample, screens for the presence of a genetic alteration of the BRAF gene (cBRAF V595E).[27] This mutation has been noted in approximately 80% of dogs with bladder or prostate cancer. This commercially available diagnostic assay has proven to be a highly sensitive means of noninvasive diagnosis for canine genitourinary cancers that harbor the BRAF mutation.[27]

Histopathologic evaluation of a tumor biopsy is considered the gold standard for diagnosis of TCC.[13–17] Biopsies may be obtained via traumatic catheterization, cystoscopic biopsy, or an open surgical biopsy.[30] Care must be taken with any disruption of a bladder, prostate, or urethral mass because of the potential for abdominal seeding.[31]

Once a biopsy sample is obtained, tumor grade, degree of invasiveness, and margin analysis (if surgically excised) are established. Most canine TCCs are reported to be grade II (36%–81%) or grade III (16%–64%) based on degree of cell differentiation, anisocytosis, and anisokaryosis, and presence of nucleoli.[1,12–17] Although the true impact of tumor grade on prognosis is unknown, increasing grade is associated with increasing vascular invasion and decreased survival.[16,17]

Imaging Options

A tentative diagnosis is made via identification of a bladder or urethral mass on abdominal ultrasound examination or other imaging, although other inflammatory and neoplastic diseases should be considered.

Plain abdominal radiography is unrewarding in the detection of TCC because the bladder silhouette is not generally distorted by the tumor. In some instances, a caudal abdominal mass, enlarged mineralized regional lymph nodes or prostate, or lytic lesions in the lumbar spine or pelvis from bone metastasis may be detected. Contrast urography provides better detail of the lower urinary system and is a useful diagnostic modality when abdominal ultrasound is not available. Filling defects from bladder tumors and/or irregularity or reduced patency of the urethra become apparent in 93% to 96% of cases.[32,33]

Abdominal ultrasonography is the most commonly relied on imaging tool to evaluate the bladder, urethra, and prostate. TCCs can have a wide variety of appearances on abdominal ultrasound, which overlaps those of other tumors, benign polyps, cystitis, and urethritis so definitive diagnosis of TCC cannot be made on ultrasonographic appearance alone.[32,33] Although useful, abdominal ultrasound is subject to limitations for monitoring response to therapy. For example, changes in bladder size and interobserver variations by ultrasound operator result in significant differences in measurements leading to misclassification of tumor responses with correlation coefficients of only 0.4 to 0.7.[34]

Cystoscopy allows visual inspection of the entire urethral lining, the trigone area, the ureteral orifices, and the bladder lining.[30,34,35] However the appearance of lesions observed cystoscopically is not diagnostic for TCC because benign tumors and proliferative urethritis/cystitis can have a similar appearance.[30,35] Cystoscopy also allows collection of pinch biopsies for histologic evaluation.

Staging

TCC staging includes routine bloodwork and urinalysis as a minimum database. Urine culture is often indicated because secondary infections are common. Thoracic radiographs are essential to evaluate for metastasis to the lungs. Caution is advised when interpreting thoracic radiographs because lung metastasis from TCC can appear as unstructured interstitial opacities, which may be incorrectly interpreted as normal aging change.[36] Abdominal ultrasound is used to evaluate for disease spread to other areas within the abdomen, such as local lymph nodes.

Staging is based on a TNM classification scheme (**Table 1**).[41] The most common metastatic sites include medial iliac lymph nodes, lungs, liver, and vertebral bodies.[1,12–17] Because most patients (61%) die from causes related to the primary tumor,[1] the true metastatic potential of TCC has not been fully elucidated.

Prognosis

Several factors have been tested for their impact on prognosis (**Table 2**). The most consistent variables seem to be related to staging, such as lymph node involvement, the presence of distant metastasis, and T3 tumors, which are all strongly associated with decreased survival (see **Table 1**).[1,13–17]

Treatment Options

Cyclooxygenase (COX)-2 inhibitory nonsteroidal anti-inflammatory drugs are recognized to be the mainstay treatment of many canine cancers including TCC.[42–45] In dogs with TCC treated with the nonsteroidal anti-inflammatory drug piroxicam, disease stabilization was noted in 53%, partial responses in 12%, and complete responses in 6%.[42–45] Similar results have been reported with the more COX-2 selective drugs, deracoxib and meloxicam.[46,47]

Table 1
World Health Organization TNM staging of canine urinary bladder TCC

TNM Classification	Description	% Affected at Diagnosis	% Affected at Death
T_0	No evidence of primary tumor	0	0
T_{is}	Carcinoma in situ	0	2
T_1	Superficial papillary tumor	2	0
T_2	Tumor invading bladder wall	78	60
T_3	Tumor invading neighboring organs	20	37
N_0	No regional lymph node involvement	84	60
N_1	Regional lymph node involvement	16[a]	40[a]
N_2	Regional and juxtaregional lymph node involvement	16[a]	40[a]
M_0	No evidence distant metastasis	86	51
M_1	Distant metastasis detected	14	49

[a] Study was unable to determine precise nature of lymph node involvement from the records.
Data from Owen LN, World Health Organization. Clinical stages (TNM) of canine tumours of the urinary bladder. In: TNM classification of tumours in domestic animals. 1st edition. Geneva (Switzerland): World Health Organization; 1980. Available at: http://apps.who.int/iris/handle/10665/68618. Accessed January 2, 2019.

Table 2
Potential prognostic factors for canine urinary bladder TCC

Negative Factor	MST (d)	P Value	Reference
N1	70 vs 234	.0001	Knapp et al,[12] 2000
Prostate involvement	71 vs 228	.001	Boria et al,[37] 2005
M1	105 vs 203	.0163	Knapp et al,[12] 2000
T3	118 vs 218	.0167	Knapp et al,[12] 2000
Sclerosis	NR	.029	Valli et al,[17] 1995
Grade II or III (vs grade I)	NR	.035	Valli et al,[17] 1995
Male gender	145 vs 358	.042	Rocha et al,[16] 2000
Platinum alone (vs platinum + anthracycline)	132 vs 358	.042	Rocha et al,[16] 2000
Cisplatin alone (vs cisplatin + piroxicam)	246 vs 309	.07	Knapp et al,[38] 2000
Grade III (vs grade II)	205 vs 365	.099	Rocha et al,[16] 2000
Lymphatic invasion	145 vs 349	.178	Rocha et al,[16] 2000
Cisplatin dose	145 vs 321	.224	Greene et al,[39] 2007
GST positive	87 vs 251	.257	Rocha et al,[16] 2000
Cisplatin vs carboplatin	203 vs 365	.439	Rocha et al,[16] 2000
DNA ploidy	NR	.58	Clemo et al,[40] 1994
P-gp positive	206 vs 263	.657	Rocha et al,[16] 2000
Serosal invasion	139 vs 302	NR	Rocha et al,[16] 2000

Abbreviations: GST, Glutathione-S-transferase; MST, Median survival time; NR, No response; P-gp, P-glycoprotein.

Chemotherapy

Many chemotherapy agents combined with a COX-2 inhibitor have been evaluated in the management of canine TCC with variable success; these include doxorubicin, cisplatin, carboplatin, and others.[37–39,48–58] At this time, chemotherapy combined with a COX-2 inhibitor (eg, meloxicam, deracoxib, or piroxicam) is considered to be the preferred initial treatment.[54] The most commonly used chemotherapy agents with efficacy include mitoxantrone, vinblastine, and metronomic or continuous low-dose chlorambucil.[59–61] Because of the variable success of chemotherapy in treating TCC, evaluation of different drugs or drug combinations is an area of active research. One recent study evaluated chemotherapy administration where the chemotherapy drug, vinblastine, was followed with a course of a nonselective COX inhibitor, piroxicam.[60] In this study, sequential administration of single agent vinblastine followed by piroxicam alone had a significantly longer median overall survival time of 531 days compared with the simultaneous administration of vinblastine and piroxicam of 299 days.[60] Possible explanations for this phenomenon include a delay in resistance mechanisms when effective treatments are administered sequentially rather than the standardly used contemporaneous administration of chemotherapy agents. Similarly, it is possible that vinblastine may sensitize the tumor or allow selection of clones of tumor cells within the tumor that would then respond to subsequent COX inhibitor treatment.[60] These results are compelling and reinforce the need for more studies to elucidate optimal treatments/treatment schedule when treating canine TCC.

Surgery

Because of the trigonal location of most TCCs and invasive nature of this cancer, surgical excision with complete histopathologic margins is not achievable.[62,63]

Additionally, TCC may be present in multifocal lesions in the bladder because of the "field effect," and implantation of tumor cells at the surgical incisions has also been observed.[31,64,65] Therefore, surgical treatment of TCC is generally not recommended.[1,13–17] For palliative measures, placement of indwelling low-profile cystotomy catheters have been used to relieve urethral obstructions with some success.[66,67]

Palliative therapies

Laser ablation of the tumor tissue as a debulking procedure can result in rapid clinical improvement.[68,69] Reported complications included stranguria, hematuria, urethral stenosis, cystitis, local tumor seeding, and urethral perforation.

Stents can also be placed into canine ureters and urethras and the application of this technique has been recently reviewed.[70–73] In one study of 12 severely obstructed dogs with urethral tumors, two-thirds were considered to have a good to excellent outcome with stent placement. Most dogs were continent after the procedure, but 17% became severely incontinent. Survival after the procedure was short, however, with a median of only 20 days.[70] Perhaps with earlier intervention improved post-procedure outcomes will be achieved.

Because of the high complication rate with either stent placement or laser ablation, these procedures are generally recommended for those clinicians with experience in these techniques.

Radiation therapy

Radiation therapy has been infrequently used in the treatment of canine TCC because the cells are considered moderately radioresistant with a high repair capacity.[74] Surgical debulking of the tumor ± intraoperative radiation followed with fractionated external beam radiation produced median survival times of 3.5 to 4 months.[15,74–77]

FELINE TRANSITIONAL CELL CARCINOMA

In cats, urinary tract neoplasms are uncommon with the exception of renal lymphoma. Approximately 60% of primary bladder cancer in the cat is TCC, which has also been reported in the feline kidney.[1,2,11] The anatomic distribution of bladder TCC is different in cats compared with dogs with the nontrigonal bladder wall being affected in 55% of cases.[11,78] Consequently, surgical options may be more beneficial in this species. Urethral stenting has been successfully performed in cats with nonmalignant urinary obstructions and reported in one cat with urethral neoplasia.[79] Other tumor characteristics and survival times are similar to the dog.[78,80]

COMPARATIVE ASPECTS OF TRANSITIONAL CELL CARCINOMA

As in several other naturally occurring canine cancers, TCC is notable for its ability to serve as a powerful model for muscle-invasive bladder cancer in humans with regards to cellular and molecular features, molecular subtypes, biologic behavior (sites and frequency of metastasis), and response to therapy.[81] Several reports exist that review the potential for dogs to reliably predict the outcome of various therapies, including immunotherapies, targeted therapies, and new combinations of conventional chemotherapy agents.[81–85] Most notable is the development of BRAF inhibitors for targeted treatment of BRAF mutant tumors. Targeted therapies such as this have proven to be highly effective in several human malignancies harboring the BRAF V600E mutation.[81,82,85] Future studies are needed to establish canine BRAF and possibly other mutations as a guide for individualized medicine in canine and human genitourinary tumors.[27,85]

REFERENCES

1. Knapp DW, McMillan SK. Tumors of the urinary system. In: Withrow SW, Vail DM, editors. Small animal clinical oncology. 5th edition. St Louis (MO): Saunders/Elsevier; 2013. p. 579–80.
2. Meuten DJ. Tumors of the urinary system. In: Meuten DJ, editor. Tumors in domestic animals. 4 edition. Ames (IA): Iowa State Press; 2002. p. 509–46.
3. Bryan JN, Henry CJ, Turnquist SE, et al. Primary renal neoplasia of dogs. J Vet Intern Med 2006;20(5):1155–60.
4. Edmondson EF, Hess AM, Powers BE. Prognostic significance of histologic features in canine renal cell carcinomas: 70 nephrectomies. Vet Pathol 2015;52(2):260–8.
5. Parekh H, Rini BI. Emerging therapeutic approaches in renal cell carcinoma. Expert Rev Anticancer Ther 2015;17:1–10.
6. Michael HT, Sharkey LC, Kovi RC, et al. Pathology in practice. Renal nephroblastoma in a young dog. J Am Vet Med Assoc 2013;242(4):471–3.
7. Montinaro V, Boston SE, Stevens B. Renal nephroblastoma in a 3-month-old golden retriever. Can Vet J 2013;54(7):683–6.
8. Seaman RL, Patton CS. Treatment of renal nephroblastoma in an adult dog. J Am Anim Hosp Assoc 2003;39:76–9.
9. Lingaas FL, Comstock KE, Ewen F, et al. A mutation in the canine BHD gene is associated with hereditary multifocal renal cystadenocarcinoma and nodular dermatofibrosis in the German Shepherd dog. Hum Mol Genet 2003;12(23):3043–53.
10. Locke JE, Barber LG. Comparative aspects and clinical outcomes of canine renal hemangiosarcoma. J Vet Intern Med 2006;20:962–7.
11. Henry CJ, Turnquist SE, Smith A, et al. Primary renal tumours in cats: 19 cases (1992-1998). J Feline Med Surg 1999;1(3):165–70.
12. Knapp DW, Glickman NW, Denicola DB, et al. Naturally-occurring canine transitional cell carcinoma of the urinary bladder. Urol Oncol 2000;5(2):47–59.
13. Henry CJ. Management of transitional cell carcinoma. Vet Clin North Am Small Anim Pract 2003;33(3):597–613.
14. Mutsaers AJ, Widmer WR, Knapp DW. Canine transitional cell carcinoma. J Vet Intern Med 2003;17(2):136–44.
15. Norris AM, Laing EJ, Valli VE, et al. Canine bladder and urethral tumors: a retrospective study of 115 cases (1980-1985). J Vet Intern Med 1992;6(3):145–53.
16. Rocha TA, Mauldin GN, Patnaik AK, et al. Prognostic factors in dogs with urinary bladder carcinoma. J Vet Intern Med 2000;14(5):486–90.
17. Valli VE, Norris A, Jacobs RM, et al. Pathology of canine bladder and urethral cancer and correlation with tumour progression and survival. J Comp Pathol 1995;113(2):113–30.
18. Backer LC, Coss AM, Wolkin AF, et al. Evaluation of associations between lifetime exposure to drinking water disinfection by-products and bladder cancer in dogs. J Am Vet Med Assoc 2008;232(11):1663–8.
19. Glickman LT, Raghavan M, Knapp DW, et al. Herbicide exposure and the risk of transitional cell carcinoma of the urinary bladder in Scottish Terriers. J Am Vet Med Assoc 2004;224(8):1290–7.
20. Glickman LT, Schofer FS, McKee LJ, et al. Epidemiologic study of insecticide exposures, obesity, and risk of bladder cancer in household dogs. J Toxicol Environ Health 1989;28(4):407–14.

21. Raghavan M, Knapp DW, Dawson MH, et al. Topical flea and tick pesticides and the risk of transitional cell carcinoma of the urinary bladder in Scottish Terriers. J Am Vet Med Assoc 2004;225(3):389–94.

22. Raghavan M, Knapp DW, Bonney PL, et al. Evaluation of the effect of dietary vegetable consumption on reducing risk of transitional cell carcinoma of the urinary bladder in Scottish Terriers. J Am Vet Med Assoc 2005;227(1):94–100.

23. Macy DW, Withrow SJ, Hoopes J. Transitional cell carcinoma of the bladder associated with cyclophosphamide administration. J Am Anim Hosp Assoc 1983;19:965–9.

24. Billet JP, Moore AH, Holt PE. Evaluation of a bladder tumor antigen test for the diagnosis of lower urinary tract malignancies in dogs. Am J Vet Res 2002;63(3):370–3.

25. Henry CJ, Tyler JW, McEntee MC, et al. Evaluation of a bladder tumor antigen test as a screening test for transitional cell carcinoma of the lower urinary tract in dogs. Am J Vet Res 2003;64(8):1017–20.

26. Borjesson DL, Christopher MM, Ling GV. Detection of canine transitional cell carcinoma using a bladder tumor antigen urine dipstick test. Vet Clin Pathol 1999;28(1):33–8.

27. Mochizuki H, Shapiro SG, Breen M. Detection of BRAF mutation in urine DNA as a molecular diagnostic for canine urothelial and prostatic carcinoma. PLoS One 2015;10(12):e0144170.

28. Nyland TG, Wallack ST, Wisner ER. Needle-tract implantation following us-guided fine-needle aspiration biopsy of transitional cell carcinoma of the bladder, urethra, and prostate. Vet Radiol Ultrasound 2002;43(1):50–3.

29. Vignoli M, Rossi F, Chierici C, et al. Needle tract implantation after fine needle aspiration biopsy (FNAB) of transitional cell carcinoma of the urinary bladder and adenocarcinoma of the lung. Schweiz Arch Tierheilkd 2007;149(7):314–8.

30. Hume C, Seiler G, Porat-Mosenco Y, et al. Cystosonographic measurements of canine bladder tumours. Vet Comp Oncol 2010;8(2):122–6.

31. Gilson SD, Stone EA. Surgically induced tumor seeding in eight dogs and two cats. J Am Vet Med Assoc 1990;196(11):1811–5.

32. Naughton JF, Widmer WR, Constable D, et al. Accuracy of three-dimensional and two-dimensional ultrasonography in measuring tumor volume in dogs with transitional cell carcinoma of the urinary bladder. Am J Vet Res 2012;73:1919–24.

33. Leffler AJ, Hostnik ET, Warry EE, et al. Canine urinary bladder transitional cell carcinoma tumor volume is dependent on imaging modality and measurement technique. Vet Radiol Ultrasound 2018;59(6):767–76.

34. Owen LN, World Health Organization. Clinical stages (TNM) of canine tumours of the urinary bladder. In: TNM classification of tumours in domestic animals. 1st edition. Geneva (Switzerland): World Health Organization; 1980. Available at: http://apps.who.int/iris/handle/10665/68618. Accessed January 2, 2019.

35. Childress MO, Adams LG, Ramos-Vara J, et al. Comparison of cystoscopy vs surgery in obtaining diagnostic biopsy specimens from dogs with transitional cell carcinoma of the urinary bladder and urethra. J Am Vet Med Assoc 2011;239:350–6.

36. Messer JS, Chew DJ, McLoughlin MA. Cystoscopy: techniques and clinical applications. Clin Tech Small Anim Pract 2005;20(1):52–64.

37. Boria PA, Glickman NW, Schmidt BR, et al. Carboplatin and piroxicam therapy in 31 dogs with transitional cell carcinoma of the urinary bladder. Vet Comp Oncol 2005;3(2):73–80.

38. Knapp DW, Glickman NW, Widmer WR, et al. Cisplatin versus cisplatin combined with piroxicam in a canine model of human invasive urinary bladder cancer. Cancer Chemother Pharmacol 2000;46(3):221–6.

39. Greene SN, Lucroy MD, Greenberg CB, et al. Evaluation of cisplatin administered with piroxicam in dogs with transitional cell carcinoma of the urinary bladder. J Am Vet Med Assoc 2007;231(7):1056–60.

40. Clemo FA, DeNicola DB, Carlton WW, et al. Flow cytometric DNA ploidy analysis in canine transitional cell carcinoma of urinary bladders. Vet Pathol 1994;31(2):207–15.

41. Walter PA, Haynes JS, Feeney DA, et al. Radiographic appearance of pulmonary metastases from transitional cell carcinoma of the bladder and urethra of the dog. J Am Vet Med Assoc 1984;185(4):411–8.

42. Knapp DW, Richardson RC, Bottoms GD, et al. Phase I trial of piroxicam in 62 dogs bearing naturally occurring tumors. Cancer Chemother Pharmacol 1992;29(3):214–8.

43. Knapp DW, Richardson RC, Chan TC, et al. Piroxicam therapy in 34 dogs with transitional cell carcinoma of the urinary bladder. J Vet Intern Med 1994;8(4):273–8.

44. Mohammed SI, Bennett PF, Craig BA, et al. Effects of the cyclooxygenase inhibitor, piroxicam, on tumor response, apoptosis, and angiogenesis in a canine model of human invasive urinary bladder cancer. Cancer Res 2002;62(2):356–8.

45. Knapp DW, Glickman NW, Mohammed SI, et al. Antitumor effects of piroxicam in spontaneous canine invasive urinary bladder cancer, a relevant model of human invasive bladder cancer. Adv Exp Med Biol 2002;507:377–80.

46. McMillan SK, Boria P, Moore GE, et al. Antitumor effects of deracoxib treatment in 26 dogs with transitional cell carcinoma of the urinary bladder. J Am Vet Med Assoc 2011;239(8):1084–9.

47. Knottenbelt C, Chambers G, Gault E, et al. The in vitro effects of piroxicam and meloxicam on canine cell lines. J Small Anim Pract 2006;47(1):14–20.

48. Chun R, Knapp DW, Widmer WR, et al. Phase II clinical trial of carboplatin in canine transitional cell carcinoma of the urinary bladder. J Vet Intern Med 1997;11(5):279–83.

49. Chun R, Knapp DW, Widmer WR, et al. Cisplatin treatment of transitional cell carcinoma of the urinary bladder in dogs: 18 cases (1983-1993). J Am Vet Med Assoc 1996;209(9):1588–91.

50. Moore AS, Cardona A, Shapiro W, et al. Cisplatin (cisdiamminedichloroplatinum) for treatment of transitional cell carcinoma of the urinary bladder or urethra. A retrospective study of 15 dogs. J Vet Intern Med 1990;4(3):148–52.

51. Ogilvie GK, Obradovich JE, Elmslie RE, et al. Efficacy of mitoxantrone against various neoplasms in dogs. J Am Vet Med Assoc 1991;198(9):1618–21.

52. Helfand SC, Hamilton TA, Hungerford LL, et al. Comparison of three treatments for transitional cell carcinoma of the bladder in the dog. J Am Anim Hosp Assoc 1994;30:270–5.

53. Mohammed SI, Craig BA, Mutsaers AJ, et al. Effects of the cyclooxygenase inhibitor, piroxicam, in combination with chemotherapy on tumor response, apoptosis, and angiogenesis in a canine model of human invasive urinary bladder cancer. Mol Cancer Ther 2003;2(2):183–8.

54. Henry CJ, McCaw DL, Turnquist SE, et al. Clinical evaluation of mitoxantrone and piroxicam in a canine model of human invasive urinary bladder carcinoma. Clin Cancer Res 2003;9(2):906–11.

55. Marconato L, Zini E, Lindner D, et al. Toxic effects and antitumor response of gemcitabine in combination with piroxicam treatment in dogs with transitional cell carcinoma of the urinary bladder. J Am Vet Med Assoc 2011;238(8):1004–10.

56. Poirier VJ, Forrest LJ, Adams WM, et al. Piroxicam, mitoxantrone, and coarse fraction radiotherapy for the treatment of transitional cell carcinoma of the bladder in 10 dogs: a pilot study. J Am Anim Hosp Assoc 2004;40(2):131–6.

57. Harrold MW, Edwards CN, Gravey FK. Treatment of bladder tumors by direct instillation of 5-Fluorouracil. Experimental observations in dogs. Invest Urol 1964;2:47–51.

58. Abbo AH, Jones DR, Masters AR, et al. Phase I clinical trial and pharmacokinetics of intravesical mitomycin C in dogs with localized transitional cell carcinoma of the urinary bladder. J Vet Intern Med 2010;24(5):1124–30.

59. Arnold EJ, Childress MO, Fourez LM, et al. Clinical trial of vinblastine in dogs with transitional cell carcinoma of the urinary bladder. J Vet Intern Med 2011;25(6):1385–90.

60. Knapp DW, Ruple-Czerniak A, Ramos-Vara JA, et al. A nonselective cyclooxygenase inhibitor enhances the activity of vinblastine in a naturally-occurring canine model of invasive urothelial carcinoma. Bladder Cancer 2016;2(2):241–50.

61. Schrempp DR, Childress MO, Stewart JC, et al. Metronomic administration of chlorambucil for treatment of dogs with urinary bladder transitional cell carcinoma. J Vet Intern Med 2013;242(11):1534–8.

62. Saulnier-Troff FG, Busoni V, Hamaide A. A technique for resection of invasive tumors involving the trigone area of the bladder in dogs: preliminary results in two dogs. Vet Surg 2008;37(5):427–37.

63. Stone EA, George TF, Gilson SD, et al. Partial cystectomy for urinary bladder neoplasia: surgical technique and outcome in 11 dogs. J Small Anim Pract 1996;37(10):480–5.

64. Jones TD, Wang M, Eble JN, et al. Molecular evidence supporting field effect in urothelial carcinogenesis. Clin Cancer Res 2005;11(18):6512–9.

65. Anderson WI, Dunham BM, King JM, et al. Presumptive subcutaneous surgical transplantation of a urinary bladder transitional cell carcinoma in a dog. Cornell Vet 1989;79(3):263–6.

66. Smith JD, Stone EA, Gilson SD. Placement of a permanent cystostomy catheter to relieve urine outflow obstruction in dogs with transitional cell carcinoma. J Am Vet Med Assoc 1995;206(4):496–9.

67. Stiffler KS, McCrackin Stevenson MA, Cornell KK, et al. Clinical use of low-profile cystostomy tubes in four dogs and a cat. J Am Vet Med Assoc 2003;223(3):325–9, 309–10.

68. Upton ML, Tangner CH, Payton ME. Evaluation of carbon dioxide laser ablation combined with mitoxantrone and piroxicam treatment in dogs with transitional cell carcinoma. J Am Vet Med Assoc 2006;228(4):549–52.

69. Cerf DJ, Lindquist EC. Palliative ultrasound-guided endoscopic diode laser ablation of transitional cell carcinomas of the lower urinary tract in dogs. J Am Vet Med Assoc 2012;240(1):51–60.

70. Weisse C, Berent A, Todd K, et al. Evaluation of palliative stenting for management of malignant urethral obstructions in dogs. J Am Vet Med Assoc 2006;229(2):226–34.

71. McMillan SK, Knapp DW, Ramos-Vara JA, et al. Outcome of urethral stent placement for management of urethral obstruction secondary to transitional cell carcinoma in dogs: 19 cases (2007–2010). J Am Vet Med Assoc 2012;12:1627–32.

72. Chung HH, Lee SH, Cho SB, et al. Comparison of a new polytetrafluoroethylene-covered metallic stent to a noncovered stent in canine ureters. Cardiovasc Intervent Radiol 2008;31(3):619–28.

73. Berent AC. Ureteral obstructions in dogs and cats: a review of traditional and new interventional diagnostic and therapeutic options. J Vet Emerg Crit Care (San Antonio) 2011;21(2):86–103.

74. Parfitt SL, Milner RJ, Salute ME, et al. Radiosensitivity and capacity for radiation-induced sublethal damage repair of canine transitional cell carcinoma (TCC) cell lines. Vet Comp Oncol 2011;9(3):232–40.

75. Walker M, Breider M. Intraoperative radiotherapy of canine bladder cancer. Vet Radiol 1987;28(6):200–4.

76. Withrow SJ, Gillette EL, Hoopes PJ, et al. Intraoperative irradiation of 16 spontaneously occurring canine neoplasms. Vet Surg 1989;18(1):7–11.

77. Molnar T, Vajdovich P. Clinical factors determining the efficacy of urinary bladder tumour treatments in dogs: surgery, chemotherapy or both? Acta Vet Hung 2012; 60(1):55–68.

78. Wilson HM, Chun R, Larson VS, et al. Clinical signs, treatments, and outcome in cats with transitional cell carcinoma of the urinary bladder: 20 cases (1990-2004). J Am Vet Med Assoc 2007;231(1):101–6.

79. Newman RG, Mehler SJ, Kitchell BE, et al. Use of a balloon-expandable metallic stent to relieve malignant urethral obstruction in a cat. J Am Vet Med Assoc 2009; 234(2):236–9.

80. Beam SL, Rassnick KM, Moore AS, et al. An immunohistochemical study of cyclooxygenase-2 expression in various feline neoplasms. Vet Pathol 2003; 40(5):496–500.

81. Sommer BC, Deepika D, Ratliff TL, et al. Naturally-occurring canine invasive urothelial carcinoma: a model for emerging therapies. Bladder Cancer 2018;4(2): 149–59.

82. Dhawan D, Ramos-Vara JA, Hahn NM, et al. DNMT1: an emerging target in the treatment of invasive urinary bladder cancer. Urol Oncol 2012;18:1761–9.

83. Zhang J, Wei S, Liu L, et al. NMR-based metabolomics study of canine bladder cancer. Biochim Biophys Acta 2012;1822:1807–14.

84. Hahn NM, Bonney PL, Dhawan D, et al. Subcutaneous 5-azacitidine treatment of naturally occurring canine urothelial carcinoma: a novel epigenetic approach to human urothelial carcinoma drug development. J Urol 2012;187:302–9.

85. Decker B, Parker HG, Dhawan D, et al. Homologous mutation to human BRAF V600E is common in naturally occurring canine bladder cancer-evidence for a relevant model system and urine-based diagnostic test. Mol Cancer Res 2015; 13(6):933–1002.

Moving?

Make sure your subscription moves with you!

To notify us of your new address, find your **Clinics Account Number** (located on your mailing label above your name), and contact customer service at:

Email: journalscustomerservice-usa@elsevier.com

800-654-2452 (subscribers in the U.S. & Canada)
314-447-8871 (subscribers outside of the U.S. & Canada)

Fax number: 314-447-8029

Elsevier Health Sciences Division
Subscription Customer Service
3251 Riverport Lane
Maryland Heights, MO 63043

*To ensure uninterrupted delivery of your subscription, please notify us at least 4 weeks in advance of move.

Printed and bound by CPI Group (UK) Ltd, Croydon, CR0 4YY

03/10/2024

01040479-0001